The Detection of New Adverse Drug Reactions

The Detection of New Adverse Drug Reactions

M.D.B. Stephens, MB, BS, MRCGP,
DRCOG, DMJ, Dip Pharm Med

with a guest chapter contributed by
J.C.C. Talbot, PhD, MSc, BPharm, MPS

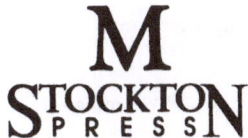

M
STOCKTON
PRESS

First published 1985

Published in the United Kingdom by
THE MACMILLAN PRESS LTD
Houndmills, Basingstoke, Hampshire RG21 2XS
and London
Companies and representatives throughout the world

British Library Cataloguing in Publication Data
Stephens, M.D.B.
The detection of new adverse drug reactions.
1. Drugs – Side effects
I. Title
615'.704   RM302.5
ISBN 978-1-349-07252-1   ISBN 978-1-349-07250-7 (eBook)
DOI 10.1007/978-1-349-07250-7
Published in the United States and Canada by
Stockton Press
15 East 26th Street, New York, NY 10010

Library of Congress Cataloging in Publication Data
Stephens, M.D.B., 1930–
The detection of new adverse drug reactions.
Bibliography: p.
Includes index.
1. Drugs — Side effects.   2. Drugs — Toxicology.
I. Talbot, J.C.C.   II. Title.
RM302.5.S74 1985   615'.7042   85–2834
ISBN 978-0-943818-33-7

Contents

Foreword

We stand on the threshold of what has been called 'the second pharmacological revolution'. During the past three decades major therapeutic advances have been made, but they may well be overshadowed by those of the rest of the century, as new molecular biochemical discoveries, and techniques for genetic engineering, permit control of viral, psychiatric, malignant and autoimmune disease. Tragically, however, this optimistic prediction is threatened by ill-advised yet widespread public fear of, and indeed hostility to, new drugs, fostered by a variety of consumer and media lobbies who have not yet understood that a chemical's therapeutic efficacy is inevitably associated with unwanted effects, particularly if used unwisely.

Many books have been written about the design of clinical trials and determination of therapeutic efficacy of drugs, but little has been published on the systematic detection, quantification and evaluation of adverse drug reactions. This process should begin, of course, with the earliest administration of a drug to man, and continue throughout its controlled clinical trials, but is likely only to identify relatively common or bizarre adverse effects. Less common, but nevertheless important, unwanted effects will be recognised only when it is prescribed for larger numbers of patients, usually after it has been marketed, and when its use, therefore, is less closely supervised.

Dr Stephens has been closely involved in the practical problems of adverse drug reaction monitoring for many years, and this book represents an important contribution to the subject which I believe will be of value to all involved in the scientific assessment of drug treatment.

Professor Paul Turner, MD, BSc, FRCP
Department of Clinical Pharmacology
St Bartholomew's Hospital Medical School
London

Preface

This book sets out to describe the problems involved in the detection of new adverse drug events both before and after a drug reaches the market and the various methods available to overcome these problems. The methods cover the collection, storage and assessment of the information. It is hoped that it will be found useful to those involved in clinical trials, whether clinician or pharmaceutical scientist. For the latter it is also hoped that he or she will find sufficient information and referenced papers to be able to set up a drug surveillance unit within a pharmaceutical company.

The withdrawal from the market of numerous drugs over the last two years has prompted changes in the regulations in many countries and, therefore, in turn has caused, and will cause, great changes within the pharmaceutical industry.

The most important change will be the realisation that equal effort and money will need to be put into both sides of the cost—benefit ratio in the clinical research of a new drug. At the time of writing, many changes are afoot and, in order to keep this book up to date, an additional chapter entitled *Update* has been included and contains the latest changes as well as references to papers that have only recently come to my attention.

I have resisted the temptation to stray into the more fascinating and controversial areas, such as the law on liability and compensation for drug injury or the history of various established adverse drug reactions, but I hope that the bibliography will have covered these gaps.

All opinions mentioned in this book are my own, unless specifically stated as being otherwise. It should not be presumed that any views or practices described here are those of the Glaxo Group or any of its subsidiary companies, unless stated.

Bishop's Stortford, 1984   M.D.B.S.

Acknowledgements

Whenever there has been need of statistical advice I have run to either D. Robinson or J. Forster at Glaxo Group Research, Ware, and evidence of this is seen in almost every chapter. Dr C. Bulpitt guided my first faltering footsteps in the world of controlled clinical trials and his influence has spread into many aspects of the book. The whole area of form design and postmarketing surveillance results from close collaboration with the late Dr J. Jackson of Clinical Data Monitoring, Glaxo Group Research, and I am deeply indebted to his help over the years.

I would not have dared to venture into the field of regulations but for the help of many people:

United Kingdom	Dr R.G. Penn
United States of America	Dr J. Dodds, Dr W.I.H. Shedden
France	Dr M. Rynikiewicz
Germany	Dr M. Hadoke, Frau G. Menck
Italy	Dr M. Pugina
Japan	Dr H. Kurihara

I am also very indebted to members of my own Drug Surveillance Department: Dr J. Talbot for his chapter on handling data, Ms M. Woods for indexing, Mrs B. Long for proof–reading and most of all to Mrs M. Rear to whom any praise for the layout and presentation of the manuscript is due.

It is also a pleasure to thank:

1. Dr Emmanueli of Farmitalia Carlo Erba for permission to publish his revised algorithm (August 1983).
2. Dr A. Ruskin for his two algorithms on drug–event association and drug–death association.
3. Dr J.A. Lewis of ICI and Elsevier Biomedical Press for permission to reproduce his statistical tables on the numbers of patients required for PMS.

4. Drs S.N. Ciccolunghi, P.D. Fowler and M.J. Chaudri for the use of the 'Ciccolunghi–Fowler–Chaudri Method'.
5. Dr B.D. Dinman and *JAMA* for permission to reproduce his tables of risk 'The reality and acceptance of risk', JAMA, 1980, **244** (11), pp. 1226–1228, © 1980, American Medical Association.
6. Dr E.S. Snell and the members of the ABPI for permission to publish the results of the 1981 survey.
7. Dr C. Stevenson for help with the design of the skin ADR form.

1
Introduction

The present situation

The first important therapeutic disaster which prompted the world to demand a better system for the detection of adverse drug reactions (A.D.R.) was thalidomide phocomelia, first mentioned in The Lancet of 2nd December 1961[1], and this was later reinforced by the practolol disaster in 1975[2]. It has been claimed that the side effects of practolol would have been discovered much earlier, had the adverse events in the early clinical trials been reported more fully[3,4]. Present pre-marketing clinical trials often fail to discover what are subsequently known to be important side effects[5,6], as witnessed by the events with Opren (benoxaprofen) and Zomax (zomepirac). The final destination of the data collected on adverse events from pre-marketing clinical trials is the licensing authority and one of these has commented that the information on adverse effects submitted by drug companies is often of poor quality[5]. Even in early clinical trials (Phase II), not all adverse effects are reported[7].

Once a drug is marketed, only about 10% of its adverse reactions are reported[8] and there is evidence that the deaths attributable to excessive use of bronchodilating aerosols were under-reported[8,9], as were the thrombo-embolic deaths due to the pill[10,12] and the practolol eye problems[11]. The poor reporting of adverse reactions for marketed drugs is not confined to the United Kingdom. America[5], France[13] and Germany[14] have reported similar problems.

In future it will no longer be sufficient for pharmaceutical companies to plan their clinical trial programme for a new drug on the basis of showing that it is efficacious and that secondarily no adverse drug reactions were noted. The cost half of the cost/benefit ratio now demands that equal effort must be put into the active search for adverse reactions as in the search for proof of efficacy.

The purpose of this book

The discovery of the A.D.R. profile of a new drug prior to marketing lies entirely within the sphere of the pharmaceutical company and, therefore, they have the responsibility for providing adequate information on a new drug. After a drug is marketed, the responsibility for extending the knowledge of the adverse reactions of a new drug spreads to all the prescribers of that drug, as well as to specific organisations set up for that purpose. The originating company, however, retains the prime responsibility for the collection of adverse reaction data from the prescribers, the assessment of its validity and informing the medical world of its evaluation.

This book reviews the methods at present used for the detection of adverse drug reactions both within and without the pharmaceutical industry and suggests improvements in methodology. The theme throughout the book is of a progressive integrated programme for the detection and evaluation of possible A.D.R. from the time a new drug first goes into man and throughout its subsequent worldwide usage.

THE COST/BENEFIT RATIO

Before treating a patient, a doctor must balance the expected benefits of a drug against its potential risks, i.e. evaluate the cost/benefit ratio. The situation is similar for the licensing authority in that their decision as to whether to allow a drug to be marketed must depend on the cost/benefit ratio for the whole population at risk. It should be the pharmaceutical industry's aim to provide the information necessary such that these decisions can be made.

To turn to the two opposing factors in the cost/benefit ratio:

    (1)   Benefits, i.e. efficacy

    (2)   Cost, i.e. the side effect liability

The benefits – measurement of efficacy

The efficacy of a drug in the treatment of a disease needs to be considered compared with three alternatives:-

(1)   No treatment and, therefore, the natural progress of the disease.

(2)   Placebo, which is the same as the above plus a psychological effect, which may produce objective benefits.

(3)   The standard treatment for that disease. If there is more than one standard treatment, then a comparison with each may be necessary.

If we presume that the healing rate for the standard therapy is greater than the natural healing rate or that induced by placebo and take as an example a healing rate of 70% for the standard therapy, we can calculate the number of patients required in the trial. In order to be approximately 90% certain of detecting a 10% difference between the standard therapy (70%) and the new therapy (60% or 80%), we would require 600 patients. If we accept the results as an adequate indication of the drug's efficacy, would this number of patients give us an adequate indication of the safety of the drug? It should certainly be able to establish the incidence of common side effects, but what chance would one have of detecting a rare serious side effect? Presuming that the side effect is identifiable as being due to the drug and that we would be satisfied in identifying one single case, we would have only a 45% chance of finding a side effect with a true incidence of 1 in 1,000 and only a 12% chance of finding two such side effects.

The cost - the statistical background to A.D.R.

With a sample size of 5,000 patients we could be more than 99% certain of finding one case of an A.D.R. with a true incidence rate of 1:1000 and, if we demand more than one case on which to base a decision as to whether this drug was safe to market, then the chances of finding them diminish rapidly, there being only a 73% chance of finding four such cases in the sample of 5,000 patients. The proviso mentioned earlier that the A.D.R. is identified as being due to the drug is, however, important. If the A.D.R. cannot be clearly differentiated from naturally occurring disease, then the problem is formidable. For instance, if the drug produced a 10% increase in a disease with a natural incidence of 1 in 1000, then - to be 95% certain of detecting this - we would require some 1,100,000 patients and for doubling of the incidence of the disease we would need approximately 16,000. For a given number of patients we can be more certain about a drug's efficacy than we can of its safety.

The reason for this situation is that a standard treatment nearly always means that it is efficacious in more than 10% of the population ($P_1 = 0.1$) and may even be effective in 50% of the population ($P_1 = 0.5$), the increase to 11% ($P_2 = 0.11$) or doubling to 20% ($P_2 = 0.2$) in the first instance and from 50% to 55% (P = 0.55) and doubling to 100% healing (P = 1.00) in the second instance - all these are relatively large figures compared with the adverse reactions that we would be interested in which might have, say, a background death rate of approximately 1:10,000 ($P_1 = 0.0001$) doubling due to treatment to 2:10,000 ($P_2 = 0.0002$) - see Table 1. The increase from 50% efficacy to 55% efficacy would need a total of 3,280 patients in the study, whilst if we wished to detect a doubling of the rate of 1:10,000 we would need 474,000. If we wished to pick up a rarity like the agranulocytosis caused by chloramphenicol, we would need 1,500,000 observations[15], and at the other end of the spectrum, if we wished to compare our new hypertensive drug against placebo and we wished to be 80% certain of finding a difference of 20mm in blood pressure (significance level 5%), we would only need 16 patients (see Table 2).

If we can satisfy ourselves as to the safety of the drug, we can assume that numbers of patients needed to do that will have been adequate for the evaluation of the drug's efficacy in the short term. It will be obvious that absolute safety is unobtainable even in the relatively short term. The problem of the changing cost/benefit ratio in the long term is even more difficult. Practolol has introduced us to the medium term A.D.R. problem with a mean time to onset of eye signs of 23 months[16], whilst the delay between the use of diethyl stilboestrol and the appearance of vaginal adenocarcinoma in the children of its recipients of at least 21 years[17], represents the long-term problem. The problem of long-term evaluation of the cost/benefit ratio has been illustrated by clofibrate where ultimately the cost has exceeded the benefits but the reasons why are not known[18,19].

It is clearly essential that maximum advantage be taken of clinical trials to establish the side effect burden of a drug and that great effort must be made to collect side effects presenting after marketing and that these must then be correctly assessed.

Table 1:   **Number of observations needed in each group to detect given change in proportion**

Power = 80%

Significance level = 5%

P_1	P_2	N
.5	.55	1640
	1.00	20
.4	.44	2490
	.80	30
.3	.33	3890
	.60	50
.1	.11	15130
	.20	240
.01	.011	168000
	.020	2700
.001	.0011	1684000
	.0020	23000
.0001	.00011	11860000
	.0002	237000

Table 2: **Number of observations needed in each group to to detect a given difference in the group means in a parallel group trial**

Power = 80%

Significance level = 5%   SD = 14 (approx)

Difference in Means	Number of Observations
2	760
5	120
10	30
15	15
20	8

THE RISKS

Since there is no way of proving the complete safety of a new drug before if comes into widespread use, it becomes a question of when do we wish to be able to define the risks. The easy answer is: as soon as possible, so that as few patients as possible are exposed to unnecessary risks. As the number of patients increases so we can define the risks with greater accuracy and then continue until the drug is marketed, when there is no longer a 100% reporting on the fate of each patient treated. Before allowing a new drug on to the market, the regulatory authority must weigh the advantages of the efficacy of the new drug, compared with the normal prognosis of the disease with known therapy, against the risks involved in marketing the new drug without full knowledge of its adverse reaction burden. At the same time the regulatory authority must decide whether they leave the detection of the more rare side effects to be discovered by the present systems or whether they should institute a major surveillance programme so that these risks may be known earlier. The decision as to how many patients should be treated before allowing a drug on to the market will depend on several factors. A relatively small number may be required for a new drug for a rare fatal disease for which there is no treatment, but several thousands may be required for a drug which needs to be taken on a long-term basis for a common chronic disease which is rarely fatal and for which there are already acceptable treatments. The regulatory authority will be influenced by the Government who in their turn will be influenced by the general opinion within Parliament which should reflect public opinion.

There have been several occasions when the reaction to the publication of an A.D.R. has resulted in the unjustified condemnation of a medication.

Oxygen and retrolental fibroplasia

The discovery in 1953 that 100% oxygen, when given to neonates, could cause retrolental fibroplasia, produced a change in practice which caused a large number of neonatal deaths from hypoxia. Cross and Bolton[20,21] suggested that there were about 200,000 deaths in England and Wales and over 180,000 deaths in the United States over the subsequent two decades. These numbers were sixteen times larger than the estimated number of babies who would have been blinded by a more liberal oxygen policy.

Pertussis vaccine and encephalopathy

The reports of neurological illness following the use of pertussis vaccine resulted in the immunisation figures for the U.K. dropping from 80% of neonates to 31%[22], and produced the largest epidemic of pertussis for 20 years[23]. 3.5% of children in the encephalopathy study had had triple vaccine within seven days, compared with 1.7% of controls. The relative risk was 2.4; if the child had previously been neurologically normal, the relative risk was 3.3, but there was no significant risk if the child had diphtheria and tetanus vaccine alone. The risk of serious impairment within seven days was 1 in 110,000 and the risk of permanent impairment was 1 in 310,000[24].

Teratogenicity of Debendox

There remain some controversies concerning A.D.R. where publicity has not helped to resolve the problem. Although on three occasions the Committee on Safety of Medicines has carefully examined all the available data on the issue of whether Debendox for the treatment of morning sickness in pregnancy has produced an increased incidence of congenital abnormalities in the offspring of mothers treated with the drug, the Committee found no evidence that there was an increased risk of foetal damage with the use of this agent[25]. The adverse publicity attached to this drug produced such a large fall in sales that it was no longer viable commercially and has been withdrawn from the market. It is the first drug victim of trial by the media.

The risks that we are prepared to take

It is very difficult to find out what risk the general public would be prepared to run for an effective drug but one can study the risks they are prepared to take in everyday life and with certain common social drugs (see Table 3).

If we examine the action that various risks have provoked, we will have an idea as to whether the public considers them acceptable or not.

Table 3 :   **The risks of common voluntary activities**

Voluntary risks[26,27,29]	Death/Person/Year (odds)	
Smoking (20 cigarettes per day)	1 in	200
Drinking (1 bottle of wine per day)	1 in	13,300
Soccer*	1 in	25,000
Car racing	1 in	10,000
Car driving* (U.K.)	1 in	5,900
Motorcycling	1 in	50
Rock climbing**	1 in	7,150
Taking contraceptive pills	1 in	50,000
Power boating	1 in	5,900
Canoeing	1 in	100,000
Horse-racing*	1 in	740
Amateur boxing*	1 in	2,000,000
Professional boxing**	1 in	14,300
Ski-ing	1 in	1,430,000
Pregnancy (U.K.)	1 in	4,380
Abortion (legal less than 12 weeks)***	1 in	50,000
Abortion (legal more than 14 weeks)***	1 in	5,900

*Based upon deaths/per million participants/year
**Based upon deaths/per million hours/year spent in sport
***Based upon deaths/per million pregnancies per year

Table 4 :   **Rare risks in life (involuntary)**

Involuntary risks[27]	Risk of death/person/year	
Struck by auto (U.S.)	1 in	20,000
Struck by car (U.K.)	1 in	16,600
Floods (U.S.)	1 in	455,000
Earthquakes (California)	1 in	588,000
Tornados (Mid West)	1 in	455,000
Lightning (U.K.)	1 in	10,000,000
Falling aircraft (U.S.)	1 in	10,000,000
Falling aircraft (U.K.)	1 in	50,000,000
Explosion pressure vessel (U.S.)	1 in	20,000,000
Release from atomic power station		
at site boundary (U.S.)	1 in	10,000,000
at 1 km (U.K.)	1 in	10,000,000
Flooding of dikes (Holland)	1 in	10,000,000
Bites of venomous creatures (U.K.)	1 in	5,000,000
Leukaemia	1 in	12,500
Influenza	1 in	9,000
Meteorite	1 in	100 billion

(1)   Fatal accidents presenting risks of 1:1000/person/year are infrequent. That immediate action is taken to reduce such hazards suggests that this level of risk is socially unacceptable.

(2)   At lethal accident levels of 1:10,000/persons/year public money is spent to control their causes.

(3)   Mortality risks of 1:100,000/person/year are still considered candidates for some action.

(4)   Fatal accidents with a probability of 1:1,000,000/person/year are not of concern to most people.

These figures show the boundaries of acceptable risk to lie between 1:1,000,000 (those associated with natural hazards) and 1:1,000, i.e. the annual per capita illness and disease risks. Society appears to accept voluntary risks with orders of magnitude greater than involuntary risks[26] (see Tables 3 and 4).

Dinman[27] points out that a country (the United States) that accepts 200,000 excess deaths a year associated with smoking and 20,000 excess deaths from not buckling seat belts will not - and to be consistent, should not pursue extreme risks posed by environmental contaminants.   More recently, there was considerable opposition to the parliamentary bill which made the fastening of front seat belts mandatory, a move which the B.M.A. had suggested would save more than 700 lives per annum and 11,000 seriously injured per annum[28].

The risks we take with drugs

To compare these figures with those of deaths caused by drugs is extremely difficult since there is gross under-reporting of the latter and, therefore, the following figures must be considered in that light and also bearing in mind the source of the figures (i.e. seriously ill patients). In the Boston Collaborative Drug Surveillance Programme 0.9 per 1000 were considered to have died as a result of drugs. The rates varied from 0 in Israel and Italy to 1.4 per 1000 in New Zealand[30].

If we consider figures for the U.K., then Girdwood[31] gives the following table:

Table 5 : **Numbers of deaths reported as possibly due to drugs in seven-and-a-half years or less**

Oral contraceptives	332	Acetylsalicylic acid	72
Phenylbutazone	217	Oxphenbutazone	69
Chlorpromazine	102	Indomethacin	68
Corticosteroids	94	Halothane	57
Isoprenaline	84	Amitriptyline	50
Phenacetin	77		

These figures, however, do not give any idea of the population at risk. The same author also gives a table based on the ratio of reports of deaths per annum compared with the number of millions of prescriptions.

Table 6 :
The ratio of reports per annum of deaths/millions of prescriptions

Sodium aurothiomalate	164.3	Indomethacin	4.4
Phenindione	30.0	Imipramine	3.6
Warfarin	28.3	Chloramphenicol	3.6
Phenelzine	17.2	Phenytoin	3.0
Oxyphenbutazone	14.3	Chlorpropamide	3.0
Tranylcypromine	13.7	Amitriptyline	2.3
Adrenaline	9.6	Trifluoperazine	2.0
Chlorpromazine	8.6	Methaqualone/diphen.	1.9
Isoprenaline	7.9	Frusemide	1.3
Propranolol	7.4	Methyldopa	1.3
Phenylbutazone	7.1	Corticosteroids	0.84
Orciprenaline	6.2		

These figures have shown the involuntary risks that patients have to run and those voluntary risks they are prepared to exchange for various pleasurable pursuits. If we accept that at lethal accident rates of 1:10,000/person/year public money is spent to control their causes and that at 1:100,000/person/year mothers warn children of the dangers of playing with fire, of drowning and of poison and some people accept inconvenience, such as avoiding air travel[27], where should we draw the line as acceptable risk with, say, a treatment with a new hypertensive drug? It has been suggested[32] that, at the time of marketing, risks of 1:100 should be known, but we must remember that this figure is not the risk of deaths but only of adverse drug reactions. It would seem that a similar figure for postmarketing surveillance is 1:1000[33] - 1 in 10,000 is acceptable[34] and this would require a cohort of 10,000 to 20,000 individuals. If a side effect is exceedingly rare, say 1:50,000, no formal system will be sufficiently cost effective to discover it.

THE NUMBER OF PATIENTS NEEDED TO ASSESS RISKS

The phrase "risks of 1:100" needs clarification. It probably refers to those distinct drug reactions for which there is no background incidence. There are two classifications of adverse drug reactions from the statistical point of view:

(1)   The adverse reaction which is clearly an adverse drug reaction and for which there is no naturally occurring background, i.e. the oculomucocutaneous syndrome with practolol. (See Table 7)

(2)   The adverse reaction which either simulates disease or produces, in
       fact, an increase in a naturally occurring disease, i.e. dry eyes
       caused by beta-blockers.   (See Table 8)

Table 7 :   **Number of patients required with no background incidence
             of adverse reactions**[35]

Expected incidence of adverse reaction	Required number of adverse reactions		
	1	2	3
1 in 100	300	480	650
1 in 200	600	900	1,300
1 in 1,000	3,000	4,800	6,500
1 in 2,000	6,000	9,600	13,000
1 in 10,000	30,000	48,000	65,000

All these tables are based on a 95% probability of success, so that our
10,000 population will give us a greater than 95% chance of having at
least three recognisable adverse drug reactions with an incidence of
1:1000 and a 95% chance of discovering two recognisable adverse drug
reactions with an incidence of 1:2000.

So if in post-marketing surveillance we have just the known incidence in
the population, i.e. control infinite, our 10,000 patients will give a 95%
chance of discovering an additional incidence of 1 in 100 where the
background incidence is 1 in 10, but a less than 95% chance of discovering
an additional incidence of 1 in 1000 when the background incidence is 1
in 1000.   (See Table 8)

Monitoring for multiple A.D.R.

The figures so far presume that one is only monitoring for one adverse
reaction, whereas in most cases we will be monitoring for an unknown
number of adverse reactions and, since we are using the 5% level of
significance, of every 100 possible adverse drug reactions examined five
adverse reactions could be expected by chance.   The world has already
been troubled with at least two probable false positives - the suggestion
of increased breast cancer with reserpine[36] and the fear of congenital
abnormalities with Debendox[25].   (See Table 9)

Table 8 : Number of patients required in drug treated group when background incidence exists[36]

Size of control	Background incidence of adverse reaction	Additional incidence of adverse drug reaction		
		1 in 100	1 in 1,000	1 in 10,000
Infinite (background incidence known)	1 in 10	10,000	980,000	98,000,000
	1 in 100	1,600	110,000	11,000,000
	1 in 1000	500	16,000	1,000,000
5 times as big as treated group	1 in 10	12,000	1,200,000	120,000,000
	1 in 100	9,000	130,000	13,000,000
	1 in 1000	700	19,000	1,400,000
Equal to treated group	1 in 10	20,000	2,000,000	200,000,000
	1 in 100	3,200	220,000	22,000,000
	1 in 1000	1,300	32,000	2,300,000

Table 9 : **Number of patients required in drug treated group to allow for examination of 100 adverse reactions**[35] (Significance P< 0.05)

Size of control	Background incidence of adverse reaction	Additional incidence of adverse drug reaction		
		1 in 100	1 in 1,000	1 in 10,000
Infinite (background incidence known)	1 in 10	23,000	2,200,000	*220,000,000
	1 in 100	3,100	250,000	24,000,000
	1 in 1000	800	32,000	2,500,000
5 times as big as treated group	1 in 10	27,000	2,600,000	260,000,000
	1 in 100	4,000	300,000	29,000,000
	1 in 1000	1,300	40,000	3,000,000
Equal to treated group	1 in 10	46,000	4,400,000	440,000,000
	1 in 100	7,200	510,000	48,000,000
	1 in 1000	2,900	73,000	5,100,000

* This is approximately the combined total population of France, Italy, Germany and the United Kingdom.

If we realise that this type of post-marketing surveillance, i.e. without concurrent randomised controls, is searching for hypotheses and not testing them and if it is accepted that nothing will be published until a hypothesis testing study is finished, then this risk is not important, except from the point of view of cost, but if, as it seems, possible hypotheses are published, we must increase the level of significance if we are to prevent more widespread apprehension (see Table 9).

These figures presume that the drug is given to the same population as has the known background incidence of the disease. It is very unlikely that the background incidence will be known in the particular subset of the population who will be prescribed the drug. Another presumption is that there will be no drop out of patients over the monitoring period.

Conclusions

Very many fewer patients are required to detect an A.D.R. which has no background incidence compared with one which mimics or increases a known disease. Many A.D.R. mimic known diseases and the means of differentiating between them often does not develop until several years have passed. If a new drug causes a modest increase (10%) in the incidence of a common disease (1 in 100 per annum), the number of patients needed for monitoring to discover this is prohibitively large[37] (250,000).

DEFINITIONS AND CLASSIFICATIONS OF ADVERSE REACTIONS

Adverse event

"Particular untoward happening experienced by a patient[38,4] undesirable either generally or in the context of the disease".

The definition used in Prescription Event Monitoring[39] is: "An event is any new diagnosis, any reason for referral to a consultant or admission to hospital (e.g. operation, accident or pregnancy), any unexpected deterioration (or improvement) in a concurrent illness, any suspected drug reaction, or any other complaint which was considered of sufficient importance to enter in the patient's notes.

Adverse reaction

"An adverse reaction is any response to a drug that is noxious and unintended and that occurs at doses used in man for prophylaxis, diagnosis or therapy, excluding failure to accomplish the intended purpose"[40]. This is a modified version of the W.H.O. definition and is the more appropriate since it excludes "failure to accomplish the intended purpose".   The United States Food and Drug Administration (1979) uses a completely different definition: "Any experience associated with the use of a drug whether or not considered drug-related and includes any side effect, injury, toxicity or sensitivity reaction or significant failure of expected pharmacological action".   This definition could be more suitable for "adverse event" than for "adverse drug reaction"[41] (see page 13). However, for the purpose of the pharmaceutical physician the following definition is preferable, since it includes all undesirable clinical events but makes no reference to inappropriate dosage.   "An A.D.R. is an undesirable clinical manifestation that is consequent to and caused by the administration of a particular drug. The clinical manifestation may be an abnormal sign, symptom or laboratory test or it may be a cluster of abnormal symptoms and tests"[42].

It is important that all adverse medical events rather than A.D.R. or side effects are collected, since the latter two terms imply that they were caused by drugs and, if the recorder is not certain if the event was caused by a drug, it would not be recorded.   The term "adverse event" is preferable   and should be used in clinical trials[4,43,44] and post-marketing[45,46].

There are seven different types of classification of adverse reaction and all are necessary for different purposes. Several different classifications are available for each type of classification. These have been chosen as the most appropriate for this purpose.

Pharmacological classification

Type A (Augmented): Those that result from an exaggeration of a drug's normal pharmacological actions when given in the usual therapeutic dose; normally dose-dependent.

Type B (Bizarre): Those that represent a novel response[47] not expected from known pharmacological action.

Causality classification

1.   **Karch and Lasagna classification**[40]

Definite: A reaction that follows a reasonable temporal sequence from administration of the drug or in which the drug level has been established in body fluids or tissues; that follows a known response pattern to the suspected drug and that is confirmed on stopping the drug (dechallenge) and reappearance of the reaction on repeated exposure (rechallenge).

Probable: A reaction that follows a reasonable temporal sequence from administration of the drug; that follows a known response pattern to the suspected drug; that is confirmed by dechallenge and that could not be reasonably explained by the known characteristics of the patient's clinical state.

Possible: A reaction that follows a reasonable temporal sequence from administration of the drug; that follows a known response to the suspected drug but that could have been produced by the patient's clinical state or other modes of therapy administered to the patient.

Conditional: A reaction that follows a reasonable temporal sequence from administration of the drug; that does not follow a known response pattern to the suspected drug but that could reasonably be explained by the known characteristics of the patient's clinical state.

Doubtful: Any reaction that does not meet the criteria above.

2. **Modified Karch and Lasagna**

The above definition needs some modification for use in pharmaceutical research. The word "definite" is too absolute as it is possible to conceive of a non-drug-related adverse event which could fit this definition, and the fact that experienced physicians find, on occasion, that they need to re-rechallenge supports this opinion. "Almost certain" is more applicable. One attribute of this definition "that follows a known response pattern to the suspected drug" would preclude its application to new drugs, so this attribute should be left out when used with new drugs. The category of "conditional" is suggested as a way of preventing the loss of previously unsuspected drug reactions which implies that all that is "doubtful" is lost. All classifications should be reviewed in accordance with any new evidence so the classifications "conditional" and "doubtful" can be combined under the heading of "unlikely".

Statistical classification

1. Specific - the A.D.R. has no known natural occurrence.

2. Non-specific - an A.D.R. which either simulates or increases the incidence of naturally occurring diseases.

Severity classification

1.   **Venulet classification**[48]

   (i)   Mild/minor - no treatment required, does not complicate significantly the primary disease, suspected drug may or may not be stopped.

   (ii)   Moderate - symptoms are marked but involvement of vital organ system is moderate. No loss of consciousness. No cardiovascular failure. Treatment or hospitalisation required, or hospitalisation prolonged by at least one day. Development of definite biochemical or structural changes could justify this classification.

   (iii) Severe - fatal or life threatening, lowers the patient's life expectancy, a severe impairment of a vital organ system, even if transient; persisting for more than one month.

The latter classification mixes two separate qualities of an A.D.R.:

   (1)   Severity, which is the quantification of the reaction symptoms, mild, moderate or severe, and are best used as grades of discomfort - these are subjective symptoms and, as such, will vary from person to person.

   (2)   Seriousness, which is an objective assessment of the importance of the A.D.R. in terms of living and dying. These elements should, therefore, be separated.

Seriousness classification

1.   Symptomatic only - worries patient not doctor. Patient stops treatment or complains.

2.   Serious - worries doctor but not necessarily patient. Doctor stops treatment.

This classification needs a more detailed description when used within the pharmaceutical industry (see page 137).

Frequency classification

The use of an adjective to describe an incidence range is quite arbitrary and will depend on the type of medical practice. The one used here is envisaged for an average general practice in the United Kingdom.

   Common   -   incidence of 10% or greater.
   Occasional -   incidence less than 10% but 1% or greater.

Rare   –   incidence less than 1% but greater than 1:1000.
Very rare   –   1 in 1000 or less; or less than 10 cases in first three
                years on the market.

Mechanism classification[49]

1. Idiosyncrasy – an uncharacteristic response of a patient to a drug
    not normally occurring on administration of this drug.

2. Hypersensitivity – a reaction not explained by the pharmacological
    effects of the drug caused by an altered reactivity of this patient
    and generally considered to be an allergic phenomenon.

3. Intolerance – a characteristic pharmacological effect of a drug
    produced by an unusually small dose so that the usual dose tends to
    induce a massive overreaction.

4. Drug interaction – an unusual pharmacological response which
    cannot be explained by the action of a single drug but may be
    caused by two or more drugs.

5. Pharmacological – a known inherent pharmacological effect of the
    drug directly related to dose.   This definition includes:

        overdose – occurring on administration of a larger than
        normally administered dose of a drug.

        unavoidable side effect – occurring with average, normal dose
        of a drug.

ADVERSE REACTION PROFILE

Ideally an adverse reaction of a drug should have a profile which consists
of the following elements:

1. Manifestation (clinical or laboratory) both subjective and/or objec-
    tive.

2. Graded both for severity and seriousness.

3. Frequency or incidence both absolute and relative to similar drugs.

4. Mechanism of action.

5. Causality.

6. Predisposing factors, i.e. age, renal function, pharmacokinetic fac—
    tors, etc.

7.   Treatment and its effect.

8.   Reversibility or sequelae.

ADVERSE EVENTS

The adverse event must be discussed in the context of the many non-drug related events in the patient's life.   There are three possibilities:

Firstly that the adverse event is one of the many minor abnormalities that occur to normal persons[50].

Secondly that the adverse event is part of a disease or is a complication of a disease, which is either that for which the drug was prescribed or a subsequent disease.

Thirdly that the adverse event is in some part caused by the treatment used for the disease and, of course, we may have interactions between any of the three.

Symptoms in healthy persons

Reidenburg[50] investigated 414 healthy students and hospital staff of Temple University, U.S.A., taking no medication, and surveyed their symptoms retrospectively using a questionnaire.   Only 19% stated that during the previous 72 hours they had experienced none of the 25 symptoms listed.   The median number of symptoms experienced per person was two.   Thirty people experienced six or more symptoms.   The symptoms listed varied from pains in muscles and joints, headaches, skin rashes and urticaria to mental symptoms and changes in bowel function, all of which have been described as adverse drug reactions.

Results of a questionnaire survey of normal patients, untreated hypertensives and treated hypertensives

The variety of symptoms that can be caused by a disease or any of its complications is vast, but, taking the specific area of hypertension, an adverse event questionnaire[51] has been used in a survey of normal subjects, untreated hypertensives and treated hypertensives[52].   The normal patients were randomly selected from a local general practice register and the untreated patients were newly referred hypertensives at the Hammersmith Hospital.   Although the survey showed that headaches, unsteadiness, lightheadedness or faintness and nocturia could actually be caused by raised blood pressure, this was so in only a proportion of those patients complaining of these symptoms (see Table 10).

It will be seen how common many of these symptoms are in all three groups and in any one person complaining of a symptom, who was on treatment, how difficult it could be to allocate it to a particular group[53].

Table 10 : Symptoms in normal persons, untreated hypertensives and treated hypertensives[52]

Symptom	Normal	Untreated hypertensives	Treated hypertensives
Sleepiness	31.4%	43.2%	51.4%**
Dry mouth	20.5%	23.7%	40.2%***
Unsteadiness on standing or in the morning	7.9%***	35.4%	33.5%
Nocturia	45.3%***	68.4%	73.2%
Diarrhoea	15.5%	25.8%	30.4% *
Depression	34.3%	44.7%**	29.4%
Blurred vision	14.7%	29.8%*	20.6%
Weak limbs	18.4%	34.0%	26.4% N.S.
Nasal stuffiness	26.8%	29.7% N.S.	– N.S.
Poor concentration	4.0%	12.8% N.S.	– N.S.
Vivid dreams	25.3%	27.8% N.S.	– N.S.
Nausea	12.0%	19.8% N.S.	– N.S.
Impotence	6.9%	17.1%	24.6% ***
Slow walking pace	9.5%***	24.2%***	37.0% ***
Waking headache	15.1%	31.3%***	15.5%
Failure of ejaculation	0	7.3%	25.6%***

Asterisks with table refer to χ^2 comparisons between one result and the result underlined in other columns.

   * $P < 0.05$
  ** $P < 0.01$
*** $P < 0.001$
N.S. Not significant.

Adverse reactions to placebo

Symptoms which are, in some part, caused by treatment must be divided
into those effects caused by the chemical constituents and those caused
by the giving of a "medication", even though the "medication" is known
not to cause side effects by its chemical nature, i.e. lactose or chalk.
The latter are normal placebo responses and have specific characteristics
which resemble those of active chemicals.

Definition

A placebo can be defined as "any component of a therapy (or control in
experimental studies) that is without specific activity for the condition
being treated or being evaluated"[54].

Commonest complaints

A review of 67 publications for unwanted or toxic side effects which
occurred during the administration of a placebo showed that drowsiness
was the most common side effect, followed by headache. Stimulation of
the central nervous system manifested as daytime nervousness or insomnia
was the third most common effect, followed by nausea and constipation[55].

Physical changes

Although the symptoms are activated via the mind they can produce
physical changes to the nose, skin, bladder, oesophagus, stomach, colon,
heart and blood vessels and kidneys[56,57,58], such as vomiting, sweating,
diarrhoea, constipation, eosinophilia, hyperacidity and skin rashes[54]. One
case has been reported of a patient meeting the definition of being
"dependant" upon a placebo[59].

Frequency of placebo reactions

The placebo tends to increase the incidence of symptoms that pre-exist
and females tend to have more frequent and severe placebo reactions than
males[60]. When placebos were administered to professional people, 58%
complained of one or more side effects and, contrary to expectations,
some symptoms decreased in the institutionalised aged when they were
given placebo[61].

Variation with age

On the whole the incidence of placebo reaction rises linearly with age[61].

Variability in type of effects

Placebo side effects, when the placebo is used as a control for an active
drug, are often similar in type to the side effects of the active drug
itself[62]: throbbing headaches after placebo in a hydralazine study;
"closed" nose after reserpine placebo[63]; diminished perception of high
tones after streptomycin placebo[64]. Once a patient on placebo or active
drug has complained of an adverse event, an observer will note that these

patients have more further symptoms than those who did not complain of the adverse event, suggesting that there is an increased interest in those patients who show change[65].

Psychological differences in placebo reactors

Lasagna and his colleagues[66] were able to show differences of attitude, habits, educational background and personality structure between the persons who consistently responded to placebo and those who did not, but that reactors were not "whiners" or "nuisances", not typically male or female, not young or old and had the same average intelligence as the non-responders. In volunteers placebos can cause effects in 66% of subjects[67] and 35% of patients[68].

Placebo pharmacology

It has also been shown that the placebo has its own pharmacology with peak effects, cumulative effects, carry-over effects and a varying efficacy, depending on the severity of the complaint being treated[69]. Placebos can relieve post-operative dental pain and naloxone blocks this effect, suggesting that the placebo acts through endorphin release[70,71].

Severity of placebo reaction

The fact that placebo reactions can be severe has been noted by several authors[58,61]. In the recent Norwegian multicentre study[72] on the comparison of timolol and placebo in inducing reduction of morbidity and reinfarction in patients surviving acute myocardial infarction, many patients were withdrawn due to an adverse reaction and were subsequently found to be on placebo.

Range of placebo reaction

In a study of more than 1,000 cases of side effects of placebo there were 35 different symptoms. The most important are listed below[73]:

Table 11:

Numbness	36 out of 72 =	50%
Headaches	23 out of 92 =	25%
Fatigue	10 out of 57 =	18%
Sensation of heaviness	14 out of 77 =	18%
Inability to concentrate	14 out of 92 =	15%
Drowsiness	7 out of 72 =	10%
Nausea	9 out of 92 =	10%
Dryness of the mouth	7 out of 77 =	9%
General weakness	5 out of 57 =	9%
Flushes	6 out of 77 =	8%

It will be apparent that it may well be impossible to tell whether a side effect, which has occurred whilst on active treatment, is due to that treatment or might have occurred if a placebo had been given instead.

2
The Methodology of the Collection of Adverse Event Data

COLLECTION OF ADVERSE EVENTS

Factors affecting collection of adverse events

In order to collect A.D.R. efficiently, it is necessary to know which factors might hinder their collection so that these can be circumvented. Between the advent of an adverse event and its final assessment as an A.D.R. the adverse event must be communicated. The factors preventing this communication are:

Failure of patient recognition

The adverse event may not be recognised by the patient for the following reasons:

(a)   No symptoms, i.e. biochemical change, hypertension, etc.

(b)   Change in mood, only recognised by relatives or friends.

(c)   Lack of intelligence or mental illness[74] (patient).

Failure of the patient to communicate adverse event to doctor

(a)   Patient does not connect the event with the drug and, therefore, does not consider it relevant.

(b)   Patient recognises the event as a possible A.D.R. but presumes that one has to put up with it.

(c)   Patient recognises the event as a possible A.D.R. and stops the drug but does not mention it to the doctor.

(d)   Patient does not inform the doctor for fear of being thought neurotic.

(e)   Poor memory (patient).

Failure of doctor to recognise adverse event as a possible A.D.R.

(a)   Doctor refuses to allow the patient to communicate the event by not giving the patient the opportunity due to a poor relationship with the patient.

(b)   Doctor listens to the patient but fails to consider possibility of A.D.R.

(c)   Doctor fails to take positive steps to look for well-known side effects, i.e. does not ask questions and/or examine patient.

Doctor recognises event as a possible A.D.R. but does not report it because of[75]:

(a)   Complacency - he thinks that it has probably been reported before.

(b)   Fear of litigation.

(c)   Guilt at causing the patient to suffer.

(d)   Ambition to collect and publish a series.

(e)   Ignorance of the mechanism of reporting.

(f)   Diffidence in reporting doubtful A.D.R.

(g)   Lethargy - too busy, etc.

The filtration of adverse events by means of protocols and forms

Bearing in mind the factors that can prevent the reporting of an adverse event to the company, steps can be taken to overcome them during any studies organised by the company, by the use of the study protocol and the forms for the collection of data. The wording of the protocol and the form design need to be appropriate to the stage in the drug's development. The overall framework necessary is outlined in Table 12.

Table 12 : Collecting adverse events at different stages of clinical studies

Stage	Adverse Events to be collected	Doctor's action (Clinical trialist)	Protocol Design	Form Design
1 Suitable for Phase 2-3-4 Studies. Double blind controlled studies.	Mild symptoms but forgotten if not prompted. Will include a lot of non-drug, non-disease events.	Not mentioned spontaneous-ly to doctor.	Adverse event reporting to be stressed and will include the wording of a standard question.	a) Patient diary card b) Patient questionnaire c) Doctor's checklist + d) Standard question
2 Suitable for uncon-trolled studies.	Mild symptoms. Remem-bered but will only be mentioned spontaneously if given the opportunity.	Doctor must give patient the opportunity to report adverse events by the use of a standard question.	Should include a standard patient question at each visit.	Adequate space for patient's reply at each visit
3 Suitable for G.P. sur-veys or uncontrolled studies.	Moderate symptoms. Remembered and men-tioned to doctor.	Doctor must be en-couraged to take full his-tory and examine patient and make clinical diagnosis.	Requests all doctors to report clinical diagnoses.	Space for clinical diagnosis.
4 Suitable for certain monitored release studies.	Moderate to severe illness.	1. Referred to hospital or second opinion. 2. Serious illness with possible sequelae. 3. Death	1. Requests all details of hospital or out-patient visits. 2. Defined illnesses. 3. Requests details.	1. Space for final diagnosis. Hospital name and address, and consultant's name. 2. Details.
5 Suitable for certain case-control studies and epidemiological surveys.	Death.	Death certificate. (unreliable as a source of diagnostic data even when certified by hospital clinicians)77	Epidemiological surveys.	Details can be obtained from Office for Census & Surveys but death certifi-cates are rarely reliable when filled in by general prac-titioners 76

This framework is not intended to be comprehensive but to give a general outline of the changes required during the development of a drug. Stage 1 represents the early part of the drug's development with relatively small, closely controlled, clinical trials. The numbers involved in each study increase with the progress through the stages, finishing at stage 5 which is suitable for postmarketing surveys involving very large numbers and may be exemplified by the asthma deaths survey[9]. The studies progress from stage 1, where there is no filtration of adverse events, to stage 2, where only the replies to a standard question and spontaneously reported events are recorded, and then to stage 3, when symptoms alone are filtered out and only clinical diagnoses reported, whilst in stage 4 G.P. diagnoses are filtered out and only those events severe enough to require hospital attention or having possible sequelae are reported. Stage 5 is the ultimate - deaths only are reported, all else having been filtered out. When a study is planned, the aim of the study must be worded so that the appropriate adverse events/diagnoses are collected and recorded.

Separation of adverse reactions from placebo reactions

Since adverse non-drug symptoms are common[50], and are not easily separated from drug-induced symptoms, both must be collected for analysis if a complete profile of adverse reactions is to be made. However, this technique can only be used in controlled studies - ideally with placebo, as well as with other standard drugs. The temptation to subtract the adverse events in the placebo group from those in the active drug group (see below) should be resisted. (This will be dealt with further in Chapter 3).

Drug group   -   placebo group   =   adverse reactions to drug

$$\begin{array}{ccc} \text{Drug-induced events +} \\ \text{Non-drug adverse events +} \\ \text{Placebo induced events} \end{array} - \begin{array}{c} \text{Non-drug events +} \\ \text{Placebo-induced events} \end{array} = \begin{array}{c} \text{drug-induced} \\ \text{events} \end{array}$$

Adverse drug reactions which are similar to common non-drug adverse events are rarely described, or investigated, sufficiently for a causal relationship for each individual event to be established. If they cannot be distinguished qualitatively, then the correct quantitative procedure is to compare them using non-parametric statistics, giving the confidence limits for the incidence of A.D.R. Small studies ($N < 30$) have little chance of separating A.D.R. from the placebo or non-drug events unless they are very common and specific to the drug[44]. Unfortunately, the situation is made worse by the fact that members of a placebo group have a tendency to "catch" A.D.R. from the active drug group and, therefore, may change a relatively specific A.D.R. to a non-specific event[56,62] (see page 15).

METHODS OF COLLECTION FOR SYMPTOMATIC ADVERSE EVENTS

The collection of all adverse events or symptoms should only be done:

(1)   where the possibility of comparing the adverse events of one group with those of another is possible, since the "background noise" of the non-drug symptoms can overwhelm the drug-induced symptoms in uncontrolled studies.

(2)   where the use of a questionnaire or checklist makes statistical comparison valid.

(3)   where they can be collected at the beginning and end of a study as a minimum.

The patient can be prompted to report all adverse symptoms if the doctor uses either a diary card, a patient questionnaire or a checklist with a standard question.   Since the majority of A.D.R. occur within the first week of drug treatment, the first visit should be then if all the minor events are to be collected.   There is a steep fall-off in recollection of minor events in young intelligent volunteers and this is likely to be greater in the elderly sick.

Patient diary card[78,79,80,81]

In those trials where a patient diary card is used for the recording of patient information, i.e. for recording daily peak flow rates in an asthma trial, it can also be used for the recording of adverse events. It is, in fact, the equivalent of answering a daily standard question. If sufficient space is allotted to the daily recording of any adverse events in sufficient detail, the diary card is likely to be unmanageably large. The large amount of unstructured data that is likely to be collected over any period longer than a few days would be difficult to handle. Daily recording of objective data with weekly recording of adverse events would make the data easier to handle without loss of important events.

An intermediate method, incorporating features of a diary card and those of a questionnaire, has been used in a large scale general practitioner study comparing demethylchlortetracycline and placebo[82]. Patients were supplied with six reply-paid postcards for recording for each day of the six months of the trial the presence of cough, spit, purulent spit, purulent nasal discharge, attendance at the doctor, work loss both with and without insurance certificate and whether trial tablets were taken. The cards included a request to indicate other medication taken and any side effects of treatment. A "record card", also reply-paid, was enclosed for immediate return, indicating occupation, smoking habits, family size, house type, work loss due to respiratory illness the previous year, and age. This card was identified, as were the monthly morbidity cards, by a code

Table 13 : Patient questionnaire

Advantages	Disadvantages
1. They can be given directly to the patient and returned directly to the organiser by-passing the prescribing doctor. Questions involving sexual behaviour can be answered more frankly than by any other method.	1. Needs great care in the wording of questions[81].
2. The involvement of the prescribing doctor can be minimal.	2. Needs considerable organisation and costs to print, distribute, collect and analyse.
3. Answers to very precise questions can be given and there is almost no limit to the number of questions posed.	3. If the questionnaire bypasses the prescribing doctor, the patient may forget to report important side effects to the doctor, forgetting that he does not see the answers to the questionnaire.
4. Confidentiality can be kept by the use of patient numbers only.	4. Questions can identify the side effects of marketed drugs but not the as yet undiscovered side effects of a new drug. This may bias a study of a standard drug against a new drug in favour of the new drug. This can be partly countered by adding an open standard question.
5. Different questions can be used for males and females.	5. Should not be used in un-controlled studies.
6. Questions can be designed for the different drugs.	
7. Is more likely to lead to the conclusion that the incidence of side effects resulting from a given drug is higher than that resulting from placebo[79].	

number. Patients whose monthly reply card had not been received by the middle of the next month were sent a reminder, which was repeated, if necessary, a month later. After three reminders, no further action was taken. The reply rate was 92%.

PATIENT QUESTIONNAIRES

The patient questionnaire is most suitable for trials where the new drug is a variant of an already standard type of drug, i.e. entirely new side effects are not expected. The Institut National de la Santé et de la Recherche Medicale has produced a useful book on the construction of questionnaires[83]. Most questionnaires ask qualitative questions with "yes" or "no" answers. However, this can be extended to a four possibilities answer: "absent", "mild", "moderate" or "severe", or a visual analogue scale[84,85,86] can be used for measuring subjective feelings. The latter has been used for measuring quality of sleep, dyspnoea[87], subjective sensation of resistance to breathing, and depression[88]. Questions need to be so worded that some require a negative answer[89] in the presence of symptoms, as this will make the patient read the questionnaire with more care and counteract any personal tendencies towards affirmative or negative answers.

It is not possible within the confines of this book to give exhaustive lists of questionnaires that have been used in clinical trials but the area has been particularly well developed in psychiatry where "soft" data has always exceeded "hard" data. Out of the familiar questionnaires for measuring depression, i.e. Beck Inventory[90], Hamilton rating scale[91], have developed various "Treatment Emergent Symptom/Event Scales" covering the possible adverse events with psychiatric drugs. Further development of these scales into the field of general medicine would be helpful but could never be relied on as the only means of eliciting adverse events.

1. DOTES - The Dosage record & Treatment Emergent Symptom Scale[92]

    Approved by the F.D.A. It is a formidable document.

    Contains classification of severity and causality.

    It is a 41-item scale with a scoring sheet and, as its name implies, relates the dosage record with emergent symptom scale.

2. Vinars' Systematic Assessment for Treatment Emergent Events[93]

    Contains 26 terms for use in psychiatry.

3. SAFTEE - Systematic Assessment for Treatment Emergent Events[94]

    Divided into two areas:

    1)   General Inquiry which focuses the patient's attention on health related experiences.

2)   Systematic Inquiry which is a modified physician's review of systems.

Also has provision for further inquiry into relevant facts concerning the event and for relevant laboratory data and physical findings.

4.   Swedish Side Effect Scale[95]

A five-point scale with operationally defined steps.

Other questionnaires specifically for appetite[96], fatigue[97], antihypertensive drugs[51] have been developed.

Checklists

Checklists consist of a list of possible side effects which the doctor goes through with the patient. They are of two kinds: (a) where the doctor reads out a series of standard questions, and (b) where the doctor interprets the side effects on the checklist, i.e. "oculogyric crises", to the patient. As such, different doctors are likely to word their questions differently. This may produce bias in a study unless the same doctor questions all the patients and even then he may word the questions differently considering the intelligence of each patient individually.

The advantages of a patient questionnaire in not using a doctor's valuable time probably outweigh the disadvantages of the additional cost and organisation needed. Neither a checklist nor a questionnaire should be used in uncontrolled studies.

A comparison between an open questionnaire and a 38 item checklist showed 15% of healthy persons had had symptoms in the previous three days when the questionnaire was used but 82% when the checklist was used, the latter figure confirming Reidenberg's figure (page 18). The parallel figure for patients who had been ill or taken medication in the previous three days was 69% for the questionnaire and 97% for the checklist. In addition, a greater severity of symptoms was associated with the questionnaire[103].

Standard questions

This is the other alternative and some of its characteristics have been mentioned. A common approach in double-blind controlled trials, as well as in other studies, is to record only "spontaneously volunteered side effects". When the list of factors (page 22) which can possibly prevent the reporting of adverse events is studied in relationship to this method, it will be seen that it has the following disadvantages as compared with with a standard question:

Table 14 : Checklists

Advantages	Disadvantages
1. Greater quantity of "side effects" given than with open question[98].	1. Needs greater care in wording questions.
2. Increased severity of side effects than with open question[98].	2. Needs considerable organisation and cost to print, distribute, collect and analyse.
3. Checklist is more likely to give higher incidence of side effects resulting from a drug than from placebo in neurotic patients[99-100].	3. As with the questionnaire, it will tend to be structured for marketed drugs and therefore biased against older drug, i.e. cannot cope with unpredictable side effects.
4. Like questionnaires, they are excellent for defining particular problems.	4. Number of side effects mentioned to the patient is more limited than with questionnaire since it involves the doctor's time.
5. As with the questionnaire, different questions can be used for males and females and the questions can be designed for the different drugs.	5. Questions involving sex may cause more embarrassment than with patient questionnaire.
	6. In depressed patients the checklist produced 5-10 times more side effects than open questions[101].
	7. Where standard questions are asked, they may be ambiguous, i.e. "difficulty with sexual function; Yes or No".
	8. Increases the incidence of irrelevant complaints[101].
	9. Relevant side effects are more likely to be detected if a checklist is not used[102].

(1)   The doctor may not give the patient the opportunity to mention an adverse event, and

(2)   The doctor assesses the spontaneously volunteered adverse event and, if in his judgment it was not definitely due to the drug, does not need to record it.

The standard question should be unambiguous and worded in such a way that it is not mistaken for a social courtesy.

Examples

(a)   "Have you noticed any change in bodily function or had any physical complaints in the past week?"[98].   This was used in a study in America in hospitalised depressed patients.   It very pointedly does not ask for any mental changes.   The wording might not be so easily understood by other English-speaking patients.

(b)   "How are you feeling?", followed by "How else are you feeling?" and finally "How does the drug make you feel?".   This was used in a study of neurotic outpatients in America[99].

(c)   "Have you noticed any new symptoms which might be related to the treatment?"[102]

(d)   "Did you experience any unpleasant effects from the medicine you took?"[104]

(e)   "Any problems?"[105]

(f)   "Has the treatment upset you in any way?"[85]

Examples (c), (d), and (f) imply that the patient makes decisions as to causality and will, therefore, vary in their interpretation of adverse events.

Two alternative standard questions are suggested:

(1)   "Have you had any medical problems since your last visit?"[100], or "Have you had any problems since your last visit?", or "Have you had any problems during the last week?"

(2)   "Have you felt different in any way since your last visit?"

The standard question is a suitable method for all clinical trials being able to be used in addition to patient questionnaires or checklist, as well as independently.   If the question is worded correctly, it should collect all drug-related events but not stimulate the production of too many non-drug related events.   If the standard question is worded to collect all events as defined by Finney as "particular untoward happening experienced by a patient undesirable either generally or in the context of the disease"[38], then it includes non-medical events, i.e. social. The problem of dealing with large amounts of social data in uncontrolled and controlled studies has not yet been solved in the drug trial context. Until the methodology of collecting, recording and analysing social events has advanced and the pattern established, firstly, for the healthy population and, secondly, for diseased groups, the definition of adverse events should be restricted to medical events.

METHODS OF COLLECTION FOR NON-SYMPTOMATIC ADVERSE EVENTS

These are the adverse events recognised by a third party, usually the doctor, but not by the patient. It will include changes in the physical findings on examination, i.e. blood pressure readings, as well as changes in laboratory investigations. The collection of data implies that it is useful and will be used. Let us take as an example the pre-marketing programme of clinical research on a new drug requiring 3,000 patients, each patient having laboratory investigations on three occasions (pre-trial value and then one intermediate value and then a terminal value at the end of the study).

The standard number of estimations to be made on each occasion is approximately 25 and includes haematological, biochemical and urinary measurements. Therefore, the total number of laboratory investigations will be a minimum of 225,000. Since the usual range given in a laboratory is based on the mean $\pm$ two standard deviations, a two tailed analysis will show in 1 in 20 of these investigations as abnormal when they have arisen by chance alone, i.e. false positives. If we presume that we are only interested in an abnormally high or low value - single tailed test - then the figure is 1 in 40, so that there will be roughly one false positive test for every two blood samples taken. In the pre-marketing programme mentioned above we should expect approximately 5,625 laboratory abnormal values by chance alone in the new drug group. The separation of these chance abnormalities from the drug-induced abnormalities will be discussed in Chapter 3.

The cost of these 25 examinations has to be considered in relation to their value in detecting drug-related problems and also whether it would be better to confine some of the standard tests to a limited number of patients and then investigate the effect of the drug on other laboratory tests. There is another possibility which is more suitable for post-marketing studies: after a specific number of patients have been closely monitored, only pre-trial laboratory estimations are performed and further tests are only performed if the clinical situation warrants them or at the end of the study.

LABORATORY INVESTIGATIONS

Choice of Investigation

The standard spread of laboratory investigations covers seven fields:

1. Liver - bilirubin, SGOT, SGPT, GGT, alkaline phosphatase

2. Kidney - urea, creatinine

3. Metabolic/electrolytes - glucose, potassium, sodium, chloride, bicarbonate, calcium, total protein, albumin

4. Red blood cells - haemoglobin, RBC, MCHC, PCV, MCV, haematocrit, platelets

5. White blood cells - total WBC, neutrophils, lymphocytes, monocytes, eosinophils, basophils

6. Urine - proteinuria, glycosuria : cells, blood, bilirubin, pH

7. Miscellaneous - ESR

These investigations are the basic safety screen and, although it may be argued that some are superfluous, i.e. SGOT and SGPT, they can be helpful in detecting laboratory errors, i.e. where one of the above is the only abnormal liver function test the fact that one is grossly raised and the other is normal would support it being due to a laboratory error. The combination of a raised GGT and an MCV greater than 92 is helpful for the recognition of patients who abuse alcohol.

In many areas of chronic or recurrent therapy it may also be important to establish the effect of a new drug on many other investigations both from the possibility of interfering with the test itself as well as altering the blood level of a particular constituent. If a multi-centre study against placebo is intended, each individual centre could "adopt" an additional investigation, i.e. thyroid function tests, so that the whole range of investigations could be covered.

Assessment of laboratory investigation

Abnormal laboratory results due to drugs can also be divided into the two types A and B, Type A forming part of a drug's normal pharmacological or toxicological action and Type B representing a novel response. Type A are usually minimal changes not evident in assessing individual records but become apparent when the statistical comparison of the mean differences between the drug group and the control group is made. This aspect will be discussed in the next chapter. Type B are usually rare, more gross abnormalities which are evident on examining individual records. These are distinct adverse events which may or may not have clinical signs and/or symptoms accompanying them. In either case the clinician's opinion is required in addition to the company's opinion. The former must be collected on the laboratory investigation form and the latter left for assessment when the data is returned to the company. There are several different methods for the collection of the clinician's opinion and the following aspects must be considered.

1.   Is an opinion necessary on each parameter on each visit in each patient? In the example (3,000 patients) mentioned earlier this represents almost a quarter of a million clinical opinions. It is also very foreign to a clinician to consider the significance of an abnormal laboratory value in a vacuum without reference to previous values or other tests affecting the same organ. This approach makes little clinical sense but has been required by a regulatory authority.

2.   The next alternative is to ask for an opinion on each individual parameter for each patient at the end of the study. This will reduce the number of opinions requested. It has advantages over the previous system in that all the results from before the drug onwards are considered.

3.   The nearest approach to standard clinical practice is to consider each organ group, i.e. all the liver tests, at the end of the trial. This reduces the quarter of a million opinions required in the earlier example to 21,000. It is also wise to ask the clinician to add a global opinion, encompassing all the organ groups, at the bottom of the laboratory investigation form.

The next aspect to be considered is the type of opinion required. For computerisation a tick or a number in a box is required but this can be limiting for the clinician. Various schemes have been used with a number of choices ranging from two to ten.

(a)   **Ten categories**

    0   =   within normal range
    1   =   abnormality probably due to primary diagnosis
    2   =   abnormality probably due to concurrent disease
    3   =   abnormality not evaluable due to concurrent medication
    4   =   probable laboratory error
    5   =   clinically insignificant deviation from normal
    6   =   also has baseline (pre-treatment) value abnormal or at limit
          or normal range
    7   =   transient abnormality resolving on continued treatment
    8   =   inadequate data for interpretation
    9   =   abnormality probably due to test drug

This system is used in the U.S.A. Full investigation by the company can be restricted to category 9. Each category excludes the possibility of others, in that only one category can be used. This has the effect of forcing the clinician to say either probably due to the drug or not.

(b) **Five categories**

    1 = clinically not significant (includes probable laboratory errors)
    2 = possibly due to a drug
    3 = consistent with disease (primary or new disease)
    4 = requires further investigation
    5 = unassessable - insufficient data

These are not mutually exclusive and five boxes are provided so that more than one can be ticked, if appropriate. Category 4 reminds both clinician and trial monitor to follow-up the case.

(c) **Four categories**

It can be argued that the clinician's opinion is only required on the question of relationship of the abnormal investigation(s) to the drug and, therefore, only this relationship is considered. These require only:

    1 = almost certain
    2 = probable
    3 = possible
    4 = unlikely

using one box and they are mutually exclusive.

(d) **Three categories**

    0 = normal value
    1 = thought to be drug-related
    2 = not thought to be drug-related

This again forces the clinician from "sitting on the fence" and this is undesirable if possible drug-related abnormalities are pushed into category 2.

(e) **Two categories**

The clinician is asked to relate the result to the normal laboratory range in his hospital.

    1 = normal
    2 = abnormal

Experience shows that many physicians do not know the exact ranges and many errors have been found on checking. It is much better to supply the computer with the normal ranges and it does a better job than the clinicians.

Timing of laboratory examinations

Normally laboratory tests are done:

1.   before the study
2.   during the study
3.   at the end of the study

Before the study

Certain levels of pre-trial investigations may be used to exclude or include patients from the study. The more exclusive these are, the less one is able to extrapolate the results of the study to the general population, but on the other hand, the fewer exclusions there are, the less powerful will be the study in finding toxic effects. The latter statement needs some explanation. In a trial of 500 patients with the trial drug and 500 in the control group, the probability of detecting a toxic effect depends on the amount of background noise in the control group (see Table 15).

Table 15   :   How power changes with background noise

Prevalence of the anomaly in the control group	Increase in the prevalence of the anomaly in trial drug group*	
	1 per 100	5 per 100
5 per 100	17 per 100	91 per 100
1 per 100	37 per 100	99.5 per 100
0.1 per 100	66 per 100	99.9 per 100

Probability (per 100) of detecting a real toxic effect (POWER) in a controlled study, the agreed risk of reaching a wrong conclusion being 5 per 100[106]

Example

If the trial drug increases the toxic effect by 1% and if the "background noise" in the control group, i.e. toxic effect, is 5%, there is only a 17% chance of finding this difference, but if the "background noise" is 0.1%, there is a 66% chance of finding it.

The background noise could be reduced by having one laboratory examination done two weeks before the study and another examination one week before the study and, if either reading was outside the normal range (the mean + two standard deviations), the patient would be excluded from the study.   This would serve to exclude all patients but those with normal function or show that patients with chronic disease are stable and would, therefore, be less likely to produce abnormalities due to underlying or incipient disease during the trial.   Unfortunately, it would also make it much more difficult to recruit patients for the study.

During Phase 2 studies there will be an emphasis on exclusions so that the small scale studies will not be embarrassed by problems other than those caused by the target disease and the trial drug, whilst the large Phase 4 studies may have very few exclusions so that the results may be extrapolated to the general population.   Phase 3 studies will take an intermediate position.

During the study

A decision on the frequency of patients' visits during a study depends on many factors including the laboratory side of drug safety.   During Phase 1 studies on volunteers, laboratory investigations will have been made after a single dose and daily after multiple dose studies.   These will usually be sufficient and in Phase 2 studies in patients the investigative screening need only be carried out after a one to two week interval.   In longer studies visits should be repeated after a further two weeks and then at monthly intervals; however, the interval will vary with the type of drug and underlying disease.   Specific laboratory investigations are often required in suspect areas discovered in animal studies or where similar drugs have had problems.   However, even where courses of treatment are short it can be advantageous to have two tests whilst on the drug so that abnormalities early in the study can be contrasted with a result near the end of the study and will help to reveal laboratory or chance errors, i.e. a single abnormal early in treatment which becomes normal whilst still on the drug is unlikely to be drug-related.

At the end of the study

The laboratory results on blood, etc., taken on the last visit whilst the patient is taking the new drug or control will not be available to the clinician until some time later.   It is, I believe, essential that all drug trials should have a post-study visit for the following reasons:

1.   To examine the patient in the light of any abnormal laboratory tests from the last "drug" visit.

2.   To examine the patient for any delayed A.D.R. or withdrawal effects and to document the dechallenge in the case of previous A.D.R.

3.   To repeat any abnormal laboratory tests.

4.   To repeat laboratory screen whilst off the drug.   Any minor
      pharmacological or toxicological changes (Type A) due to the drug
      can then be seen to be reversed and help to confirm or reject the
      hypothesis that changes seen were drug-related and not due to
      disease progression.

The quality of life[107]

In those cases where chronic disease demands chronic therapy, the
cost/benefit ratio from the patient's point of view rather than the doctor's
can be assessed as the quality of life[108]. As mentioned on page 22, a close
relative or friend may be in a better position to assess some aspects of the
effect of the A.D.R. on the patient. The assessment can be recorded using
a Quality of Life Impairment Scale[109] which covers 20 areas and yields a
score of 0 to 32. The chapter on this subject in C J Bulpitt's Randomised
Controlled Clinical Trials covers this area very well (see bibliography).

SUMMARY

At each clinic visit, after the normal social pleasantries, if any necessary
objective measurements can be made it will allow time for the patient to
relax and give them the opportunity of mentioning any adverse event which
has been troubling them (spontaneously volunteered A.D.R.). If nothing is
forthcoming, then a standard question should be asked, preferably before
the patient has re-dressed, if undressing was necessary for the objective
measurement. In addition, a self-answering questionnaire may be handed
to the patient at the end of the consultation for the patient to fill in,
either in a waiting area or in their own home, but it is not a substitute
for the preceding open question. Checklists should only be used when
detailed description of a specific A.D.R. is required in comparative studies
and should not be used when non-specific A.D.R. are being hunted.

Any adverse objective measurements will require the clinician's comment
unless it is obvious from the action he takes. The protocol should contain
the words to be used as the standard question and instruction on the use
of any questionnaire needs to be given. The need for the clinician's opinion
on adverse objective measurements needs to be stated.

3
The Assessment of Adverse Medical Events

ASSESSMENT OF ADVERSE EVENTS

Once the decision has been taken as to the type of adverse event to be collected, a form should be designed for the recording of the data (see Chapter 8). Where the data is recorded by the presence or absence of a stated event (i.e. questionnaire or checklist) and the trial is a large controlled trial, it is necessary to compare the two drugs statistically rather than to try to assess each event as to its causality by the drug. Where the event is more than the transient appearance of a mild to moderate non-serious symptom, then a judgment needs to be made as to its causality and this applies to both controlled and uncontrolled studies. It is very rare that a drug can be indicted as the "complete and definite cause" of a particular adverse event without any reservations and almost as rare to be able to clear a drug of being a factor in an adverse event. The causality is, therefore, a question of opinion.

When clinical pharmacologists assessed adverse reactions submitted to them by physicians, they frequently disagreed with the physicians and each other in their assessment[110-114]. If one physician is given only a brief summary of an adverse event and case history and another has the full data available, disagreement may occur in approximately half the cases but, when both physicians have all the available data, the disagreement falls to less than one in five[113]. For the assessment of an adverse event by one who does not have complete access to the patient and their records, an intermediate form is required to make certain that all relevant information is collected.

The relevance of the different factors which need to be considered to establish a causal link in adverse reactions has only been discussed in the literature in recent years. The different factors which complicate adverse reaction assessment are the following:

(1)   Recently introduced drugs about which little is known.

(2)   Multiple drug regimens.

(3)   Drug withdrawal or dosage reduction.

(4)   Possible drug interactions.

(5)   Non-drug therapy producing adverse reactions.

(6)   Diagnostic tests and procedures producing adverse reactions.

(7)   Underlying and intercurrent illnesses.

(8)   Time delay between drug administration and occurrence of adverse event.

(9)   Common spontaneous events or transient episodic events unrelated to disease or drugs.

(10)   Irreversible events.

(11)   Tolerance or desensitization to the drug.

(12)   Specific treatment for an A.D.R. clouding dechallenge.

(13)   Prophylactic treatment clouding rechallenge[115].

In 1978 Dangoumau and his colleagues considered the responsible factors and found they came under three main headings[116,117].

(a)   Chronology - evolution.

(b)   Clinical - paraclinical.

} Intrinsic factors

(c)   Bibliography - extrinsic factor

and the first two they further sub-divided:

(a)   Chronology - evolution

        Criteria 1 : chronology of the event.
        Criteria 2 : response to stopping treatment
        Criteria 3 : rechallenge after stopping treatment

(b)   Clinical and paraclinical

        Criteria 4 : clinical symptomatology/manifestation
        Criteria 5 : other possible explanations

Criteria 6 : the patient's past history or terrain
Criteria 7 : complementary examinations

Grouping the criteria 1 to 3 together they gave chronology-evolution a score:

1st degree being doubtful
2nd degree being plausible
3rd degree being very likely.

and similarly for the criteria 4 to 7.

These factors they considered as intrinsic as opposed to the extrinsic factors which are the known factors about the drug, i.e. the bibliography, and these they also graded.

1st degree : no reference to the adverse event has been found.

2nd degree : publications are rare and uncertain.

3rd degree : the bibliography suggests that a causal relationship is probable and the criteria for this were that one of the following situations must exist.

(a)   Similar events had been numerous and/or are well documented beyond reasonable doubt.

(b)   The adverse event has been the subject of a statistical study or of an experiment to demonstrate its pharmacological mechanism.

(c)   The event is "known" or "classic" and does not justify any research.

Combining intrinsic and extrinsic factors with their degrees there were nine classes: 1 - 1, 1 - 2, 1 - 3, 2 - 1, 2 - 2, 2 - 3, 3 - 1, 3 - 3, which could be used as scores which added together gave a 5-level scale (2 - 6). Details of this method of A.D.R. assessment have been given in some length since it forms a good standard against which others can be measured.

Numerous authors have given different grades of causality and this will be referred to on page 55. The grading given below is from the definition recommended by Karch and Lasagna[118] adapted by Bennett and Lipman[49]. Once again this has been chosen as a standard since it has relatively clear cut definitions for each grade.

Degree of certainty of the relationship between drug and tissue reaction:

- (a)   definite
- (b)   probable
- (c)   possible
- (d)   coincidental
- (e)   negative

Definite

(1)   A reaction that follows a <u>reasonable</u> temporal sequence from administration of the drug

OR

in which the drug level has been established in body fluids or tissue.

(2)   That follows a <u>known response pattern</u> to the suspected drug.

(3)   That is <u>confirmed</u> on stopping the drug (dechallenge).

(4)   Reappearance of the reaction on repeated exposure (rechallenge).

Probable

(1)   A reaction that follows a reasonable temporal sequence from administration of the drug

OR

in which the drug level has been established in body fluids or tissue.

(2)   That follows a known response pattern to the suspected drug.

(3)   That is confirmed on stopping the drug (dechallenge).

(4)   That could not be <u>reasonably explained</u> by the known characteristics of the patient's clinical state.

Possible

(1)   A reaction that follows a reasonable temporal sequence from administration of the drug

OR

in which the drug level has been established in body fluids or tissue.

(2)   That follows a known response pattern to the suspected drug.

(3) Could have been produced by the patient's clinical state or other modes of therapy administered to the patient.

Conditional

(1) A reaction that follows a reasonable temporal sequence from administration of the drug

OR

in which the drug level has been established in body fluids or tissue.

(2) Does not follow a known response pattern to the suspected drug.

(3) Could not be reasonably explained by known characteristics of the patient's clinical state.

Doubtful

Any reaction not meeting the above criteria.

It will be apparent when the words underlined in these definitions are studied that considerable variation is possible in their interpretation. This would not be important if there was only a single candidate for the cause of the adverse event but, as has been stressed already, there are usually alternative drugs, procedures or disease, etc., as candidates, and frequently more than one of these could have equal claim to being causal in the grades "probable" or "possible". In order to distinguish between possible causes more grades are required and this finer gradation can be done by giving weighted scores to different questions. The grading "conditional" was added so that A.D.R. to new drugs not being able to qualify for a higher grading, due to the lack of knowledge about its response pattern, should not be lost. However, the inadequacies of this grading system become apparent when one considers that a new drug may not have acquired a "known response pattern" and yet satisfy all the other criteria for "definite".

Ideally, the responsible clinician, a clinical pharmacologist and perhaps a specialist in the field of the adverse event would sit down with all the available data and hopefully reach a consensus opinion. This is obviously not feasible except on very rare occasions. The alternative is to have an agreed standardised approach such that, when used by different experts, it gives a reproducible result similar to that given by the consensus opinion[113]. Various standardised approaches have been put forward either in the form of tables or algorithms, covering most of the points already mentioned (see Table 17). An algorithm has been defined as a set of well defined rules for the solution of a problem in a finite number of steps[119]. The criteria demanded of a method of assessment for the pharmaceutical industry are slightly different from those of other users and are:

1. Sensitivity and specificity - the ability to distinguish between two possible drug candidates.

2. Validity - the agreement between the algorithm and a consensus of opinion.

3. Reproducibility.

On the whole, time and money are available to collect all available information. The increased information warrants a more extensive algorithm with greater sensitivity and specificity. Time is not a limiting factor. The different algorithms were designed for several different circumstances and vary in their length and detail so that a further breakdown of their variation is necessary for their evaluation.

ASSESSMENT OF CAUSALITY - ELEVEN DIFFERENT APPROACHES

1. **N. Irey (U.S.A.)**[120,121]

    The first authoritative discussion of the relevant factors to be examined in order to establish a causal relationship, with definitions of degrees of certainty was published by Irey in 1972. It was based on experience gained at the Registry of Tissue Reaction to Drugs which is located at the U.S. Armed Forces Institute of Pathology and is, therefore, slightly oriented towards a pathological classification. It is not in the form of a questionnaire nor does it have a branched logic decision format. It was not written as an operational algorithm but the definitions can be used to assign causality.

2. **F. E. Karch and L. Lasagna (U.S.A.)**[118]

    This algorithm is based on a yes-no table but the individual questions are too broad for use as a sensitive tool. The validation compared the results of an investigator using the algorithm with the consensus of three experienced clinical pharmacologists and obtained a 71% agreement. It could be suitable in a purely clinical setting but not for use in the pharmaceutical industry, i.e. a yes-no answer to "known reaction to agent" could only be used some years after a drug is marketed. A modification of this algorithm was made by doctors from Sandoz Ltd., Switzerland, using a yes/no answer to 6 questions[122].

3. **J. Dangoumau, J. C. Evreux and J. Jouglard (France)**[116]

    This algorithm has already been referred to and is set in the form of a table with each criteria weighted. The main criteria are divided into "intrinsic" referring to the event and the patient and "extrinsic" which refers to knowledge of the drug. The greater attention given to varying degrees of evidence concerning the history of the drug makes this more suitable than the previous methods for use in the pharmaceutical industry but it was the least accurate when compared with methods 2, 6 and 7. When 58 cases out of 781 were judged as probable using this algorithm, subsequent follow-up showed that 35 of these side effects were subsequently described in the literature[123].

4.   **J.C.P. Weber (U.K.)**[124]

This is used by the Committee for the Safety of Medicines and is presented in standardised form for use with a computer. However, it is based on the amount of information available on the "yellow card" and is, therefore, suitable when only limited information is available. This is suitable for use in the industry if a primary form is used which is short and simple with a secondary form requesting more data requiring a more elaborate algorithm but it is not suitable for distinguishing between several   candidates.

5.   **F.D.A. Form (U.S.A.) - Jones, J.K. :**
      The F.D.A.'s Division of Drug Experience[125]

This is in the form of an algorithm with standardised questions and is suitable for computerisation. Only six standardised questions are used and it would not be sufficiently sensitive for use within the pharmaceutical industry. Obviously designed to match form FD 1639 for collection of adverse reaction data and is suitable when only information from the FD 1639 is available.

6.   **S. Blanc, P. Leuenberger, J.-P. Berger, E. M. Brooke**
      & J. L. Schelling (Switzerland)[111]

Three main criteria are used: time sequence, response pattern and role of underlying disease, and each are graded 1 to 3, the various combinations leading to five possible degrees of probability. There are no standardised questions or branched logic decision format. The validation showed a low level agreement between any two observers. It was not designed to detect new drug reactions.

7.   **M. S. Kramer, J. M. Leventhal, T. A. Hutchinson & A. R. Feinstein**
      (U.S.A.)[42,126,127]

This uses 57 standardised questions with a branched logic decision format and can be computerised. Weighting of questions varies from -1 to +1. The validation is extensive and non-experts agreed with a consensus of three experts in 80 to 83% of cases. A comparison of four experienced clinicians and four first-year interns showed a dramatic effect on level of inter-observer agreement with the experienced clinicians but little effect on the interns' agreement. This algorithm is suitable for use in the industry when full information concerning the adverse event is available but since the weightings only vary from -1 to +2 it lacks specificity.

8.   **J. Venulet, A. Ciucci & G. C. Bernecker (Switzerland)**[128]

This is designed by the staff of Ciba-Geigy and uses 27 standardised questions but does not use a branched logic decision format. The questions are weighted in multiples of 5, from +30 to -25. It also includes a visual analogue scale for causality. The validation of this method was done by Ciba-Geigy physicians, each form being assessed by an evaluator who is a physician with experience of the area of pathology in which the adverse reaction falls. The information available for the validation team was obtained by the use of forms and was "often more extensive" than that collected by the W.H.O. drug monitoring system or by the National Drug Monitoring Centre. The validation process was a comparison of the results of the Evaluator, using the non-weighted questionnaire and then allotted one of the four causality boxes, with a consensus of four evaluators using the weighted questionnaire with agreement in 61% of cases. However, since the information available was limited the consensus of opinion of the four company physicians might not have agreed with a consensus of three clinical pharmacologists with access to all the available data. A full description of this method is given in Assessing Causes of Adverse Drug Reactions (see bibliography).

9.   **C. A. Naranjo, V. Busto, E. M. Sellers, P. Saunder, I. Ruiz, E. A. Roberts, E. Janacek, C. Domecq & D. J. Greenblatt (Canada)**[129]

This uses 10 standard questions with weighting varying from +2 to -1 but without the use of a branched logic decision format. The question concerning previous knowledge of the drug "Are there conclusive reports on this reaction?", "Yes" scoring +1, "No" 0, "Do not know" 0, is insufficiently sensitive for use within the industry since "conclusive" is not defined. Validation compared the consensus of three experts and six observers (2 physicians and 4 pharmacists) and percentage agreement ranged from 79% to 84%. Several different methods were used to establish validity including comparison with method 7.[130].

However, it is difficult to see how only 10 questions can lead to a differentiation between concurrent drug therapy when the time sequence is dealt with by "Did the adverse event appear after the suspected drug was administered?", "Yes" +2, "No" -1, "Do not know" 0. There is no investigation as to whether the time sequence is appropriate for the adverse event.

10.   **A. Emanueli and G. Sacchetti (Italy)**[131]

This algorithm was developed especially for use in large scale phase III and phase IV trials by doctors from the Carlo Erba company. The answers to eight questions are limited to "yes" and "no" without any weighting. There are some internal inconsistencies in the algorithm. The second question "The possibility that clinical state or therapies may explain the event can be ruled out" ; a negative answer allows only a relationship of either "unrelated" or "doubtful possible". This would be too crude a distinction to decide between either two drug candidates or a drug reaction and naturally occurring disease.

11.   In an endeavour to create an algorithm/table which met my own personal needs, I have designed a decision table/questionnaire. The demands I made were:

    1.   That it should be sensitive and specific enough to separate different drugs.

    2.   That any bias should be in the construction of the method and minimal bias in its application.

    3.   That it should make me consider all the factors concerned.

    4.   That it could be applied to drugs in the pre- and post-marketing periods.

    5.   That it should be used for the middle range of A.D.R.:

        (a)   Most serious A.D.R. - these would be submitted to an external consultant of renown in the particular field involved.

        (b)   The common - symptomatic, minor events which can be assessed statistically but where there is limited information for an algorithm.

        (c)   The middle range - neither (a) nor (b).

It is published here merely as an example of a different approach to the problem. It has yet to be validated (pages 49-54).

12.   **Other drug regulatory authorities**

Drug regulatory authorities other than the C.S.M. and the F.D.A. use different criteria to define causal relationship. Australia defines "certain, probable, possible and unclassified"[132], whilst Sweden uses six criteria similar to those proposed by Venning[133] for literature assessment:

(a)   data from rechallenge.

(b)   a pharmacological basis for the adverse reaction.

(c)   immediate acute adverse reactions.

(d)   local reactions at the site of administration.

(e)   a first report of reactions with a new route previously recognised with ancillary method of administration.

(f)   the repeated occurrence of rare events.

(g)   suspected adverse reaction in an anecdotal series arising mainly or entirely with doses at the top end of the range normally prescribed.

for classifying anecdotal reports to regulatory authorities.

Mention must be made of one further algorithm for use in special circumstances. The Treatment Emergent Symptoms (page 28), i.e. adverse events occurring during treatment can cause a problem in psychiatric studies where the patient often has many similar symptoms before starting the drug, some of which may become worse during drug treatment, despite improvement in their psychiatric state. The exacerbation may be caused by the drugs used. Maistrello et al[134] have used an algorithm in this context with depressed patients. They use a severity scale of 0 to 3 for the unwanted symptoms and a depression scale of 0 to 3 based on the Hamilton Rating Scale for depression. A simplified version of the algorithm is shown below.

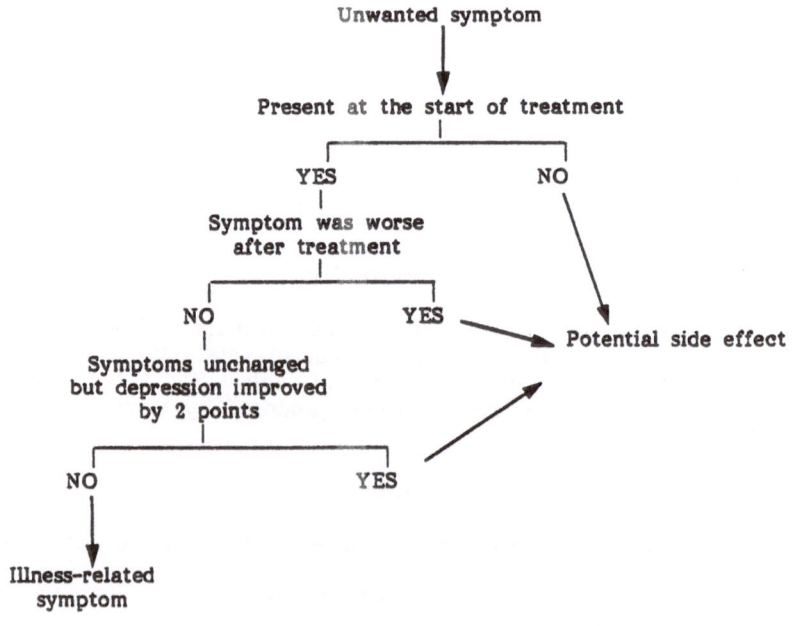

ADVERSE EVENT SCORING

There are six factors and each has a variable basic score between 1 and 10:

1-4 are against it being due to the drug.
5 and 6 are neither very much for or against it being due to the drug.
7-10 are in favour of it being due to the drug.

Since descriptions cannot fit all the circumstances exactly the score can be moved up or down 1 value. If a factor cannot be assessed due to lack of data it should be scored 5.

Alternative drug candidates should also be scored using this table.

Table 16a

FACTOR 1 : HISTORICAL EVIDENCE (Maximum score is 10)

Previous Reports (Add 1 if published) (Add 1 if some well documented)	Type of Adverse Reaction		Not on market	On U.K. Market <3 years	On U.K. Market >3 years
	Type A Pharmacological mechanism	Type B Occurrence known with other drug of same class			
NO REPORTS or they are "UNLIKELY"			5	3	1
ONLY "POSSIBLES"	Known +2 No hypothesis −2	Known +1 Not known −2	6	5	4
One or two "PROBABLES" (if more, add 1)			8	7	6
One or more "ALMOST CERTAIN"	Known +1 No hypothesis −1		9	9	9

Table 16b

FACTOR 2 : TIME TO ONSET

TYPE A   →   PHARMACOLOGICAL MECHANISM   →   TYPE B

Description	Score
Very unusual for the event	1
	2
	3
Time to onset rather unusual for this event	4
Time to onset not known	5
Only rough estimate of time to onset? Acceptable? — Event so unusual, onset time not known	6
Just within time to steady state or about acceptable. — Within wide normal limits for the event (months)	7
Well within time to steady state or acceptable timing — Within the normal limits for this event (weeks)	8
Within time to peak levels or exactly correct timing — Exactly correct timing for this event (<one week)	9
No other simultaneous drugs, i.v. drug. Onset <5 mins — Type 1 allergy. Immediate onset. (<one hour) No other simultaneous drugs	15

If adverse event started before drug administration but became worse whilst on drug, subtract 2 from score

Table 16c

FACTOR 3 : EVOLUTION OF EVENT AND DRUG WITHDRAWAL

	Score
A usually reversible reaction but continues despite stopping the drug	1
Event disappears despite continuing the drug. Tolerance to drug unlikely	2
Event already improving when drug stopped, improvement continues	4
Treatment and stopping drug simultaneously. Improvement might be due to treatment OR no information after onset of adverse event.	5
A definitely irreversible event OR event disappears despite continuing the drug. Tolerance to ADR occurs	6
Drug stopped. No treatment given. Unusually slow, fast, or slight improvement on stopping drug	7
A possibly irreversible event which continues despite stopping drug	8
Drug dose reduced. No treatment given. Improvement occurs	9
Drug stopped. No treatment given. Disappearance exactly correct for this event (no exact time given -1)	10

Table 16d

FACTOR 4 : RECHALLENGE – IF NOT PERFORMED ADD 5

Description	Score
No response – dose of duration similar to original – no other change in treatment	0
	2
Original reduction in dose and rechallenge equals re-establishment of original dose – no response	3
Lower dose than original or shorter duration of treatment – no response	4
Difficult to judge due to changes in underlying disease – no response	5
Difficult to judge due to changes in underlying disease – some response	6
Original reduction in dose and rechallenge equals re-establishment of original dose – increase in event.	7
Other drugs continued – identical response on rechallenge, or Patient says return of symptoms with each dose	8
Rechallenge with smaller dose – SOME response but not identical, or No other drugs, no change in treatment – identical response on rechallenge – derechallenge not mentioned	9
No other drugs, no change in treatment – identical response on rechallenge (If response on stopping rechallenge exactly correct for drug involved +2)	10

Table 16e

FACTOR 5 : ALTERNATIVE (DISEASE) CANDIDATE

	Score
Patient has a history of similar event without drug involvement or event typical of common complication of underlying disease or common new disease	1
Event typical of rare complication of underlying disease or rare new disease	2
Event possibly due to complication of underlying disease or new disease	3
Changes in other drugs/treatment/disease/circumstances could be the cause	4
Insufficient information given to judge	5
Situation confused by multiple therapies/diseases but they are unlikely cause	7
No change in other drugs/treatment/diseases/circumstances. Unlikely due to underlying disease or new disease	8
No other drugs given. Unlikely due to underlying disease or new disease	9
No other drugs given. Not known with any underlying or new disease	10

Table 16f

FACTOR 6 : ODDS AND ENDS

Further investigation, laboratory, biopsy, post-mortem – if none done or non-contributory add 5

	Score
Very much against drug involvement	2
No help at all	5 — Interpolate where necessary
Investigations strongly in favour of drug involvement	8
Reaction at site of application only	Additional score +10
Patient has had exactly similar reaction with a previous drug	Additional score +3

Scores

Unlikely	<30
Possible	30–36
Probable	37–40
Almost certain	>40

Should be reported with date and drug with scores

i.e. – 7.7.1983 – test drug – 6, 4+1, 3, 2, 5, 5+3 = 29 = Unlikely
   – name

If two drugs are both rated as possible causes, the one with the highest score becomes probable

Table 16 : Methods for assessment of adverse events

	1	2	3	4	5	6	7	8	9	10	11	12
Branched logic (format or questionnaire)	No	Yes	No	Yes	Yes	Yes	Yes	Yes	Yes	Yes	Yes	Yes
Validated	No	Yes	No	No	No	Yes	Yes	Yes	Yes	Yes	No	No
Score weighted	No	Yes	Yes	No	No	No	Yes	Yes	Yes	No	Yes	No
Number of questions (maximum)	6	-	18	10	4	11	57	27	10	8	60	6
A. Temporal sequence	Yes	Yes	Yes	Yes	Yes	Yes	Yes	Yes	Yes	Yes	Yes	Yes
B. Estimate of drug level	Yes	Yes	Yes	No	Yes	Yes	Yes	Yes	Yes	Yes	No	No
C. Dechallenge	Yes	Yes	Yes	Yes	Yes	Yes	Yes	Yes	Yes	Yes	Yes	Yes
D. Rechallenge	Yes	Yes	Yes	Yes	Yes	Yes	Yes	Yes	Yes	Yes	Yes	Yes
E. Alternative aetiology	Yes	Yes	Yes	Yes	Yes	Yes	Yes	Yes	Yes	Yes	Yes	Yes
F. Previous experience of drug	No	Yes	Yes	Yes	No	No	Yes	Yes	Yes	Yes	Yes	Yes
G. Site of reaction	No	No	No	No	No	No	No	No	No	No	Yes	No
H. Patient's adverse reaction history	Yes	No	Yes	No	No	No	No	Yes	Yes	Yes	Yes	No
I. Clinical pattern	Yes	No	Yes	Yes	No	Yes	Yes	Yes	Yes	No	Yes	No
Categories of causality:-												
1. Definite/certain/causative	5	5	3	3	4	5	4	5	4	5	4	6
2. Probable	Yes	Yes	No	No	Yes	Yes	Yes	Yes	Yes	Yes*	Yes	Yes
3. Possible	Yes	Yes	Yes	Yes	Yes	Yes	Yes	Yes	Yes	Yes	Yes	Yes
4. Coincidental (questionable Sandoz)	Yes	Yes	Yes	No	No	No	Yes	No	No	No	No	Yes
5. Remote/doubtful/unlikely	No	Yes	No	Yes	Yes	Yes	Yes	Yes	Yes	Yes	Yes	Yes
6. Negative/unrelated	Yes	No	No	No	No	No	No	No	No	Yes	No	Yes

*a further possibility of "almost definite" is inserted between "probable" and "definite"

Key

1. N. Irey, 1972 (page 44)
2. Karch & Lasagna, 1977 (page 44)
3. J. Dangoumau, 1978 (page 40)
4. C.S.M., Weber (page 45)
5. F.D.A., J. Jones, 1979 (page 45)
6. S. Blanc, 1979 (page 45)
7. Kramer et al, 1979 (page 45)
8. Venulet et al, 1980 (page 46)
9. Naranjo et al, 1981 (page 46)
10. Emmanueuli & Sacchetti, 1980 (page 46)
11. Stephens' Table (page 49)
12. Sandoz modification, 1978

CONCLUSIONS

All eleven algorithms and tables are very different, using different formats, questions and definitions. Six algorithms have been validated by comparing the use of the algorithm with a consensus of opinion. Comparison of four of the algorithms (numbers 2, 3, 6 and 7) showed disagreement three times out of four[135,136] in one survey, and another survey of the same algorithms showed that perfect agreement was only obtained for one case in every five[137]. Analysis in the former survey showed that number 6 (Blanc et al) was the most accurate but the least reproducible. Number 7 (Kramer et al) was the simplest to use but the most affected by suggestibility, while number 3 (Dangoumau et al) was the most reproducible and the least accurate[138]. Accuracy was measured by five different methods, all of them comparing each algorithm with various combinations of the other three algorithms. However, the nearest we can get to the truth is probably the result of a rechallenge and its subsequent dechallenge. If possible ADR were chosen at the time of dechallenge for suitability for rechallenge and the algorithm applied before the re-challenge, the results of the algorithm could be compared with the results of rechallenge, but this method has not yet been used.

In the comparison of the four algorithms it was found that in 53 of the 64 asessments in which they failed to agree, the criterion of "alternative cause" was responsible for the difference of opinion[138]. There was information on chronology of appearance, alternative cause and literature data in over 95% of the cases but details on dechallenge in only half of the cases and on rechallenge in only 4.3%. It was found in the comparison of the four algorithms that there were five major criteria:

(1)   literature search.

(2)   time course of appearance of adverse reaction.

(3)   dechallenge.

(4)   rechallenge.

(5)   alternative cause.

The weighting that should be given to each criteria was discovered by the use of multilinear regression analysis of 47 cases and the subsequent weightings tested on 15 other cases. The authors commented that the test sample was not adequate and that strictly multilinear regression analysis should only be used for numerical variables[139] but that further research should overcome these problems. Until the problem of variable weighting is solved, there is no one ideal algorithm. In the interim period the Venulet algorithm is probably the most useful for use within the industry when only minimal data is available, but the Kramer algorithm is probably more sensitive when there are alternative candidates and a large amount of data but has an insufficient range of weightings. When a previously unknown adverse reaction to a new drug is possible, a very large amount of detail is acquired by the pharmaceutical company and opinion is sought from several experts. In these cases it is probable that a consensus of opinion is preferable to any algorithmic analysis.

The clinician in charge of the patient is the best source of information on the adverse event and on the patient, whilst the pharmaceutical company is probably the best source of information on the drug. Therefore, the form used to collect information from the clinician must be designed with the use of an algorithm in mind, i.e. specifically enquiring as to any alternative candidate: "Could the original condition or other illness have accounted for these symptoms?" (see Forms 1 and 2, appendix pages 216 and 217).

Assessment of an A.D.R. by use of an algorithm may need to be repeated several times, the first assessment taking place soon after the event and the final assessment when every abnormality has returned to normal or reached a plateau and all information is gathered in[140,141,142].

Clinical assessment

The algorithm will give a causality rating to the adverse event changing it to an adverse reaction with a qualifying adjective in front varying from "an almost certain adverse reaction" to "an unlikely adverse reaction" or "negative adverse reaction". The whole will then have to be clinically assessed in its setting. The variety of responses is infinite and each case will be considered individually as regards its implications. However, one aspect deserves special consideration.

Beneficial adverse events

Although this sounds like a contradiction, one patient's adverse reaction may be another patient's treatment, i.e. hypotension was found to be a side effect of beta-blockade. Prichard converted this into one of beta-blocker's greatest assets - effective anti-hypertensive therapy[143]. Even an adverse reaction seeming to have no redeeming features, like the deleterious effect of anti-inflammatory non-steroidal drugs on renal function, can be utilised to a patient's benefit[144].

Statistical assessment

Symptomatic adverse reactions - questionnaires and checklists: the answers regarding adverse events are that they are present or absent, i.e. binary data, and are not amenable to analysis of variance or co-variance where the data is assumed to be normally distributed. The binary data are submitted to non-parametric tests such as χ^2 or Fisher's exact probability tests. The parallel test to analysis of variance for normally distributed data is for binary data multiple logistic regression[145].

ASSESSING LABORATORY DATA FROM LARGE SCALE STUDIES

Aims

(i)   To find the overall effect of the drug on each parameter.

(ii)   To try to separate individual true drug-related abnormalities from those arising by chance.

Overall effect of drug (group assessment)

This is usually a straightforward statistical exercise of comparing the mean differences (before drug and after drug) test drug compared with control. However, not all parameters have a Gaussian distribution and some require logarithmic transformation to produce the correct distribution and others cannot be manipulated into a suitable form.

Although there may be no statistical difference between the effects of the two drugs on the mean differences of a parameter before and after the drugs, it is still possible for there to be large changes in a few patients on drug A which are balanced by slight changes in many patients on drug B. One way of assessing these large changes is to compare how many patients change from being normal to abnormal and vice-versa. However, normality as represented by the normal range is arbitrary and may be different in each hospital laboratory[146], and derived from an unrepresentative sample of the population. Ideally, all laboratory estimations should be performed in a single central laboratory. Commonly, the normal range is taken as the mean $\pm$ 2 standard deviations and should have been calculated using healthy non-patients.   The computer, given the normal range (more correctly - the reference range[147]), can classify the results in several ways.

(a)   Below, above or within normal range.

(b)   Changes (before drug - after drug) greater than a fixed percentage of the normal range or various percentage changes from the baseline value.

(c)   Values going outside various extended ranges.

(d)   All cases where there is more than one related parameter outside the normal range (i.e. SGOT and alkaline phosphatase).

(e)   All changes beyond a fixed limit of clinical significance, i.e. platelets $< 100,000$.

(f)   All patients' records where laboratory abnormalities are marked by the investigator as possibly/probably due to drug.

(g)   Where there are intermediate recordings during the trial, there are further possibilities to identify:

   (i)   transient changes (normal before and after, but abnormal in between)

   (ii)   establish trends - where intermediate values are increasing.

Method (a)

This will produce the number of patients, above (A), below (B) or within the normal range (N) for before and after drug and a shift table can be constructed.

Figure 1

Post-drug

		A	N	B
Pre-drug	A	5	8	9
	N	6	3	3
	B	2	1	2

+

Scanning the figures on either side of the diagonal can give an immediate impression as to the shift of results during the trial but a statistical comparison can also be made between the number in squares NA, BA, BN (increases) and squares AN, AB and NB (decreases) or a comparison between drugs or the number of increases and decreases.

Method (b)

The two drugs can then be compared by making a table of those with significant increases (greater than 50%), those with significant decreases (greater than 50%) and those with neither:

	Drug A	Drug B
No. with significant increase		
No. with significant decrease		
No. with no significant change		

or a histogram can be drawn of the number of patients with a 0 to 10% increase, 11 to 20% increase, etc., and similarly for decreases. A visual comparison of the histogram of the new drug and its control may be helpful. A statistical comparison can also be made.

Method (c)

The normal range is the mean ± approximately 2 (1.96) standard deviations for those parameters with a Gaussian distribution and 1 in 40 of the investigations is likely to be abnormally high or low by chance. In the example given in Chapter 2, **page 32,** there could be 5,625 chance abnormalities and obviously each of these cannot be fully investigated. However, if we take the mean ± 3 standard deviations as an extended range, the chance abnormalities are reduced to 338. If the range is extended still further to mean ± 4 standard deviations, then the figure is reduced is 6 per 100,000. This is a manageable number to examine and will pick up gross abnormalities.

Methods (d) to (g)

These can be used to pick out records which need individual assessment.

Summary

In large controlled studies there needs to be a statistical comparison between laboratory abnormalities with the test drug and those with the control drug, and this may include:

1.   Comparison of the mean differences between pre-treatment values and those done at the end of the study.

2.   Comparison of the number of patients who have shifted from low or normal values to high values (and/or vice versa) with some investigations.

3.   Comparison of numbers of abnormalities beyond extended ranges.

4.   Comparison of numbers of abnormalities with more than 50% increases of the baseline value.

5.   Comparison of numbers of abnormalities beyond a fixed limit.

6.   Comparison of numbers of transient abnormalities.

Individual assessment of certain abnormalities will be necessary:

1.   All those abnormalities considered as possibly or probably drug-related by the clinician.

2.   All those abnormalities beyond fixed limits.

3. All those cases where there are two or more abnormal values in an organ group.

4. All records showing an adverse trend in any parameter.

5. Those abnormalities beyond diminishing extended ranges where there are no controls in a study. A "before and after" statistical comparison is all that is possible and any changes due to drug will be confounded by any changes in underlying and new disease occurrence over time.

Individual assessment

The individual assessment may be carried out by the clinical trialist and/or by the company physician. If the data is to be presented either to a regulatory authority or as a paper, then it is advisable that the clinician responsible for the patient with the adverse event gives his opinion. The company physician will also need to assess these cases both for internal company reports, as well as for regulatory authorities, but they must be assessed without knowing whether the patient has been taking the test drug or its control. Sufficient information should be available for the use of an algorithm or decision table.

An alternative method of assessing laboratory data from large scale multi-centre clinical trials has been put forward by personnel from Ciba-Geigy.

The Ciccolunghi/Fowler/Chaudri Method[148]

The data was first screened and classified by a computer programme. Certain parameters were given arbitrary levels:-

haemoglobin : (1) increase or decrease less than 1 gm/100 ml
(2) increase or decrease of 1 - 2 gm/100 ml
(3) increase or decrease of 2 gm/100 ml or more.

haematocrit : change of $\pm<5\%$, ±5 to 10%. $\pm>10\%$

white count : more than 10,000; 5,000 to 10,000; 4,000 to 5,000; less than 4,000 cells/mm^3

platelets : more than 150,000; 100,000 to 150,000; 50,000 to 100,000; less than 50,000/mm^3

liver function tests and blood urea nitrogen : normal or above normal

serum glucose : above or below normal range

Detailed study was restricted to white counts less than 4,000 cells/mm^3 and platelet counts less than 100,000mm^3.

Table 18 : Classification of laboratory abnormalities by the Ciccolunghi/
Fowler/Chaudri method [148]

Category	Criteria used for assignment
1.1 Spontaneous Variation or	1. Abnormality present for a maximum of 1-2 visits which was either temporary despite continued treatment or occurred on the last visit only and was minimal. A progressively increasing abnormality over 3-4 visits was never considered to be spontaneous variation. 2. No relevant unwanted effects, other laboratory abnormalities or concomitant disease. 3. No relevant concomitant medication. 4. No comment or action by investigator.
1.2 Laboratory or Recording Error	1. Usually a single aberrant value or, if more than one, evidence of centre effect. 2. No relevant unwanted effects, other laboratory abnormalities or concomitant disease. 3. No relevant concomitant medication. 4. No comment or action by investigator.
2. Minimal Change of No Probable Clinical Significance	1. Abnormality represents such slight deviation from the norm that it is obviously of no clinical significance. 2. No relevant unwanted effects, other laboratory abnormalities or concomitant disease. 3. No relevant concomitant medication. 4. No comment or action by investigator.
3. Relevant Concomitant Disease or Operation	1. Relevant concomitant disease (recorded by investigator and/ or evidenced by pre-treatment abnormality in another laboratory test) or operation present at time of abnormality. 2. Any unwanted effects or laboratory abnormalities present must confirm this impression. 3. No relevant concomitant medication. 4. Confirmatory comment or action by investigator.

4. Possible Drug Effect
 	
   4.1 No relevant concomitant medication taken.
 	
   4.2 Relevant concomitant medication taken
	1. Abnormality progressively increases during trial.
	2. Relevant unwanted effects and other laboratory abnormalities present.
	3. Confirmatory comment or action by investigator. Treatment should not be prematurely discontinued for laboratory abnormality unless relevant concomitant disease or operation present.
	4. Abnormality, other than minimal, present at the last visit only.

5. Probable Drug Effect	1. Abnormality progressively increases during trial. 2. Relevant unwanted effects and other laboratory abnormalities present. 3. No relevant concomitant medication taken or disease present. 4. Confirmatory comment or action by investigator. Treatment may be prematurely discontinued by investigator for this reason.

Each abnormality was then examined in the light of all available information by two Ciba–Geigy physicians according to the classification shown in Table 18.

It should be noted that for an abnormality to be considered as possibly or probably due to a drug, the abnormality must progressively increase during the trial, relevant unwanted effects and other laboratory abnormalities must be present and there must be confirmatory comment or action by the investigator. The paper by Ciccolunghi, Fowler and Chaudri is worth reading in full.

Pfizer have also produced a system[149]. Each abnormality was considered probably drug-related unless it fell into one of the following:

Category No. 1:   The baseline value was abnormal.

Category No. 2:   The deviation from normal was so small as to be clearly insignificant.

Category No. 3:   One or more abnormal values which returned to normal with continued therapy.

Category No. 4:   There was a single unconfirmed abnormal value.

Category No. 5:   There was a documented laboratory error.

Category No. 6:   There was evidence of a concurrent illness which was likely to cause the abnormality.

Category No. 7:   The abnormality might be due to concomitant drug usage.

Summarising laboratory investigation results

The results of the statistical comparisons must now be examined for their clinical significance. If twenty comparisons have been made, then one abnormality will be expected by chance alone (at $P < 0.05$), so a decision needs to be made as to whether any significant differences (at $P < 0.05$) are due to the drug or have occurred by chance. Confirmation can be sought either externally or internally. External confirmation is by examination of a separate database or by repetition of the study. Since many regulatory authorities demand that certain studies be performed in the country concerned, the chance of comparing results may arise. Internal confirmation is sought by:

(a)   checking the animal data to see whether any related abnormality has been reported,

(b)   checking the data from volunteer studies,

(c)   checking the adverse event database to see if there are any clinical counterparts to the laboratory abnormality,

(d)   checking the other laboratory parameters reflecting damage to the same organ or change in function.

Where there is a significant increase $(P < 0.05)$ in the number of minor events in the drug group compared with the placebo group, study of the individual cases may reveal an A.D.R. pattern or the lack of it. A scatter of the minor event throughout a study rather than concentrated in the first week would suggest a non-drug pattern. Other symptoms or laboratory abnormalities associated with the minor event may indicate several different clinical patterns and these subgroups can be compared in the drug and control groups. Finally, a comparison of the clinician's opinion on the abnormal events and laboratory abnormalities with the opinion of the pharmaceutical physician should reveal a similar pattern.

Summary

Algorithms have not yet advanced sufficiently so that any of them can be recommended for universal use. In the case of important new adverse reactions, full investigation followed by a consensus of opinion between the clinician, the pharmaceutical physician and a specialist in the field of the adverse event with the final decision lying with the latter, is probably as near to the truth as we are likely to reach. Further advances in the development of algorithms may come from the use of analogue scales (10cm line) for the main questions already outlined in the published algorithm and then for these main questions to carry weighted marks according to their importance. Assessment of laboratory data cannot be left to a statistical assessment of the means of the comparative groups. With the aid of a computer all likely abnormalities can be highlighted and detailed assessment restricted to these.

4
The Pre-marketing Establishment of the Side Effect Profile of a New Drug

Figure 2:

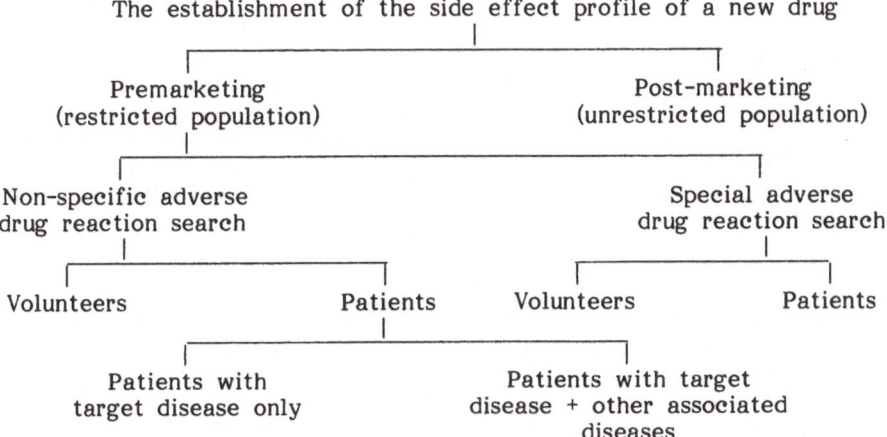

The establishment of the side effect profile of a new drug

Premarketing
(restricted population)

Post-marketing
(unrestricted population)

Non-specific adverse
drug reaction search

Special adverse
drug reaction search

Volunteers   Patients   Volunteers   Patients

Patients with
target disease only

Patients with target
disease + other associated
diseases

PRE-MARKETING STUDIES

Non-specific adverse drug reaction search

This is the search for adverse drug reactions which is undertaken for all drugs and excludes the special search for particular adverse reactions which might be foreseen from prior information.

An A.D.R. may manifest itself either by subjective symptoms or objective findings or a combination of both.

(a) **Subjective symptoms**

The early Phase 2 studies should aim to pick up the minor events which are fairly common (see Chapter 2), so that, if a particular event is shown to be more common in the drug group than in the placebo group, the later Phase 3 studies can be planned with this in mind.   Most minor events are described inadequately by clinicians, i.e. "headache", but if they are recognised early in the clinical trial programme, a specific questionnaire or form can be designed to obtain a full description as described on page 17.   If the minor event has some special characteristics, then its drug relationship can be recognised once the drug is marketed and the drug will not be stopped unnecessarily.   The questionnaire or form must, therefore, try to identify the particular clinical characteristics of the event. Secondly, the background characteristics of the patients suffering the event must be identified with the hope that a susceptible sub-group can be identified as being more at risk, i.e. the elderly, atopic, etc. Further investigation of these patients may also throw light on the mechanism of action.   Rechallenge, when it is ethical and the patient has consented, is of vital importance in establishing the drug/event relationship and should be encouraged in the protocol.   The effect of treatment of the event can frequently confound the effect of stopping the drug so the latter should precede treatment whenever possible.   Minor events are usually completely reversible on stopping the drug but it will be helpful if the speed of reversibility can be ascertained.

(b) **Objective findings**

This is usually covered by the standard laboratory investigation scheme but it is of special importance when considering the effect of the drug on the course of any chronic diseases which may be present in addition to the primary disease.   In these circumstances, it is important to measure the effect of the drug on the chronic disease and the parameters usually used for its diagnosis and prognosis.

Rarity of serious A.D.R. in volunteers

Serious A.D.R. are extremely rare in volunteers[151,150] according to the experience in the U.S.A. with only one drug-related sequela in one volunteer out of 29,162 subjects used over 12 years and only one clinically significant medical event occurring every 26.3 years of individual subjects' participation.   Minor adverse reactions are not uncommon and help towards the detection of similar adverse reactions in the clinical trials by alerting the trial designer to potential problems.

The place of women in Phase 1 studies

A study of the proportion of young women taking part in all phases of pre-marketing clinical trials for two drugs showed that they were under-represented in Phase 1 and Phase 2 studies and approximately equally represented in Phase 3 studies when compared with their proportionate use after marketing[152]. The reason for this is that the current F.D.A. guidelines proscribe administering new drugs to pregnant women and also those who might become pregnant, and specifically state that women of childbearing potential should be excluded from large scale clinical trials until the F.D.A. Animal Reproduction Guidelines have been completed.[153] These guidelines are designed to protect the potential offspring of these women. Animal testing should advance in pre-marketing programmes such that women can take part equally in Stage 3 studies but there are other reasons for excluding such women from Phase 1 and 2 studies. The presence of a few pre-menopausal women suffering from pre-menstrual tension could increase the background noise in the control group and, if distributed unevenly between the two drug groups in controlled studies, could give misleading A.D.R. data. The other reason is that the new drug must be shown not to be an enzyme-inducing agent lest the volunteer/patient on the contraceptive pill should become pregnant whilst on the new drug.

Difference between adverse events in volunteers and patients

Adverse events occurring in volunteers need to be considered quite separately from those occurring in patients and should not be added to the adverse drug reaction file for the following reasons:

(a)   **Due to absence of disease**

The volunteer does not have the disease which the drug can correct and, therefore, there may be an exaggerated pharmacological reaction in volunteers which would not occur in patients or would occur to a lesser extent, thus producing either objective effects or subjective effects[154].

(b)   **Due to incorrect dosage**

The dosage used may be outside the subsequent recommended therapeutic range due to differences between volunteers and patients[153,154].

(c)   **Due to different formulation**

Some of the volunteers may have been given a different formulation from that marketed later on.

(d)   **Due to different age, intelligence and psychological make-up**

Excluding the absence of disease, the volunteers are likely to differ from the patients who subsequently have the drug. In the U.K., volunteers are likely to be either university students or staff from the pharmaceutical company and are likely to be of greater intelligence and younger than the patients, having a more scientific background and perhaps a different psychological make-up[155,156].

(e) **Due to different relationship with clinical trialist**

The relationship between the volunteer and the person responsible is frequently that of a junior (the volunteer) to a senior (the clinical trialist) and this could affect the reporting of adverse events. Because of these differences between patients and volunteers, it has been advocated that more use should be made of volunteer patients[157,158].

Possible improvements in ADR collection in volunteers

It is, however, important that maximum use be made of the opportunity to collect adverse reactions efficiently. This may be improved by:

(1) Use of an anonymous questionnaire in controlled studies on possible sexual effects.

(2) The use of a follow-up question 24 hours after a single dose study.

(3) Standard question - the use of a standard question in all studies, i.e. "Have you noticed any physical or mental changes during the study?"

(4) Natural inhibition - various measures may be necessary to prevent the natural inhibition of the volunteer in reporting symptoms which might lead his senior to consider him "neurotic". These could include:

   (a) Collection of adverse reactions to be the job of relatively junior staff.

   (b) The publication of the fact that non-medical clinical study assistants had taken an oath of confidentiality.

   (c) The use of an anonymous written report by the volunteers after a study.

(5) Rechallenge - the more frequent consideration of rechallenge using placebo and active drug in volunteers with non-serious symptoms only.

Patients (Phase 2 and Phase 3)

These studies will progress from the use in the first patient with the target illness through small controlled studies to relatively large scale comparative clinical trials. Some Phase 3 studies will be relatively small studies in sub-groups of patients who have the target illness and other chronic conditions such as diabetes, renal failure, etc. All the protocols should specify how adverse events are to be collected and followed up. The methods used will vary according to the type of study.

Figure 3: CLINICAL STUDIES

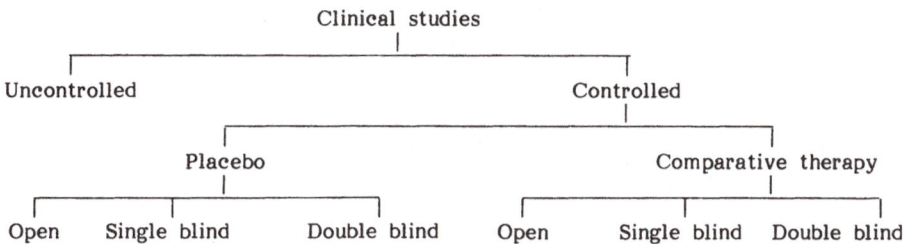

Clinical studies

Uncontrolled   Controlled

Placebo   Comparative therapy

Open   Single blind   Double blind   Open   Single blind   Double blind

UNCONTROLLED STUDIES

These may vary from the use of the drug by a physician in a single patient resistant to other therapy to relatively large scale dose-titration studies. All these studies should be governed by a protocol. All patients must be accounted for and detailed records kept.

Difficulties in attribution

From the point of view of adverse drug reactions, these studies pose several problems not found in controlled studies:-

(1)   Without a control the adverse events, which are symptoms alone and which can occur in normal persons without drugs, often cannot be attributed to the drug.

(2)   Since the type of patient admitted to the study is often not tightly controlled by a protocol, patients are entered having diseases or complications other than the target disease, giving rise to the difficulty in deciding whether an adverse event is due to the natural course of the concurrent disease (or complication) or to the drug.

(3)   Concurrent therapy is often permitted in these uncontrolled studies and, therefore, attribution of adverse events to the trial drug may be difficult.

Regulation of uncontrolled studies

At one end of the scale we have all the problems of an adverse event as it occurs after marketing with very little knowledge of the drug's adverse reaction profile. An unaccountable fatal outcome occurring in an early uncontrolled study may, quite unjustly, be attributed to the drug and all further studies stopped or delayed. The practice of allowing physicians involved in controlled studies to use the drug in a parallel uncontrolled study must be strictly limited and the physician must be prepared to monitor the patients as strictly as if in a formal controlled study. All adverse medical events, no matter how trivial, must be documented and the pharmaceutical company notified without delay of any serious reaction. This can be done either by a specifically designed record card (see Appendix, page 230) which is returned at regular intervals or by the use of a standard adverse events form type 1 or type 2 (see Appendix, pages 216 & 217) which is returnable immediately after the event has occurred. The latter has the advantage that the event report is not delayed until the main trial form is returned.

CONTROLLED TRIALS

Protocol

The protocol needs to consider all aspects of the clinical trial and it is useful to run through a checklist[159,160,80] to make certain that all the essentials have been considered. The following are the questions concerning adverse reactions that should be considered when writing the protocol.

Aim

Does the aim of the study accurately describe the purpose of the trial as far as adverse reactions are concerned?

Patient selection

Does the selection of patients bias the study as far as adverse reactions are concerned?

(a) Have patients who have previously had one of the trial drugs been excluded? If not, how will they be dealt with? There is more likely to be a problem in comparative controlled trials in chronic diseases where the alternative drugs are the new drug and the standard therapy. A patient who already has had the standard therapy without any problem is very unlikely to have an ADR in the study, whilst the patient who has developed an ADR whilst previously on the standard therapy will be excluded from the study. The statistical analysis of the trial results can weight the effect of previously having the standard against not having had it. Exclusion of these patients from the study could have a serious effect on trial recruitment. The record card must, therefore, have a space with the phrase "Has the patient ever had any of the trial medications? If so, with what result?"

(b) Has the background noise been reduced to a reasonable level? (see page 36).

(c)   Does the choice of clinical trialist or hospital bias the selection of patients as far as type, severity or resistance to treatment of the target illness?

(d)   If the target illness is chronic, will the clinical features and relevant laboratory investigations be shown to be stable prior to the study?

(e)   Are the inclusion and exclusion criteria pitched at the right level so that the trial results can be extrapolated to a reasonable population of patients on the drug, i.e. females of childbearing age, etc.[153].

Trial design

(a)   If the study is not double-blind, will the lack of blindness bias the production of adverse events in favour of one of the trial drugs?

(b)   Will the known A.D.R. of the trial drugs unblind the study? If so, how will this problem be overcome?

Concurrent therapy

(a)   What concurrent therapy should be permitted or forbidden?

(b)   Is sufficient provision made for recording of concurrent therapy on the record form?

Adverse events (symptomatic)

(a)   Have the adverse events to be collected been defined? (see page 24)

(b)   How are the adverse events to be collected:

   (i)   Diary card?

   (ii)   Questionnaire with or without analogue scale?   Has the questionnaire been validated[161]?

   (iii)   Checklist?   and/or

   (iv)   Standard question?   Is the wording in the protocol?

   (v)   Other?

(c)   Does the protocol require the clinical trialist to investigate fully all adverse events, including seeking the aid of specialists where necessary?

(d)   Does the protocol request the physician to make any interim diagnosis or drug attribution before breaking the drug code?

(e)   Does the protocol allow for a sample of blood to be taken for drug levels in the case of all serious adverse events?

(f)   Does the protocol inform the clinical trialist that all serious adverse
        events <u>must</u> be notified immediately to the company?

(g)   Do the record forms allow sufficient space and require sufficient
        details for assessment of all types of adverse event?   (see appendix
        page 230)

(h)   Does the protocol request full follow-up on patients who have stopped
        a trial drug due to an adverse event, i.e. dechallenge, or who have
        a laboratory abnormality or an adverse event at the last visit whilst
        on the drug?

(i)   Does the protocol require full details of treatment of any adverse
        event to be recorded?

(j)   Does the protocol request the consideration of rechallenge where
        ethically justified?

(k)   Who is to assess the causality of the adverse event?   Clinical trialist?
        Company physicians?   Clinical pharmacologist? Consultant specialist?
        All?

(l)   How are the adverse events to be analysed and compared?   Clinically
        only?   Statistically?   If the latter, how?   **(see page 57).**

Adverse events (asymptomatic)

(a)   Do the laboratory and other objective investigations cover the field
        of potential adverse reactions[162]?

(b)   How is the handling of patients with asymptomatic abnormal
        laboratory investigation to be dealt with[163,164]?

            (1)   by repeating tests?
            (2)   by further confirmatory tests?
            (3)   by clinical examination?
            (4)   by dechallenge?
            (5)   by rechallenge?

(c)   How are   the laboratory   examination results   to be asses-
        sed[107,165,166]?

            (i)   according   to the normal laboratory range   as normal or
                    abnormal (above/below)?

            (ii)   by the clinician and/or the company doctor?

            (iii)   clinically as well as statistically?

(d)   Will the samples be analysed centrally in a multi-centre trial? If analysed in the hospital where the trial takes place, has the pathologist been approached?

Drop-outs

How are drop-outs to be investigated/followed-up to make certain that the cause was not drug intolerance?

(a)   Is there a financial disincentive for the trialist to follow-up drop-outs, i.e. drop-outs not paid for?

(b)   Is there provision for following up patients who change general practitioner or move, so that they may be contacted for long-term follow-up?

(c)   If the study is long-term, have arrangements been made with N.H.S. Central Register in Southport for patients to be flagged so that deaths will be identified[166].

Third-party "interference"

Have sufficient arrangements been made to ensure co-operation with the management of the patient during the trial but outside the confines of the trial?

(a)   Provision for notification of trial with request to general practitioner for co-operation.

(b)   Provision for possible emergency admission to another hospital.

(c)   Recording of the use of over-the-counter products by the patient.

(d)   Provision of a card for the patient, giving details of the trial and a contact telephone number/address, requesting information from any doctor consulted.

General

What is the probability that the trial will fulfil its aim as to the adverse effects, i.e. what is the size of the type II error?

(a)   What incidence of adverse reactions (95% confidence limits) appearing with only one of the comparative drugs could be detected?

(b)   What difference in incidence of adverse reactions in the trial drug compared with the control could the trial detect?

(c)   Has it been agreed that adequate space will be given to the reporting of ADR in any subsequent papers[167], including statements as to the power of the study.

(d)   Will all patients who have been randomised and taken even a single tablet be analysed and accounted for, as far as adverse reactions are concerned[165].

RECORDING ADVERSE EVENTS IN CLINICAL TRIALS

From the point of view of recording adverse events they can be divided into two types: minor and important events.

The reasons for this differentiation into two categories - minor and major - are the following. It is unusual that minor symptoms can be causally related to the drug on an individual basis; however, they can be grouped together and their incidence compared statistically in the two drug groups. The clinicans are only likely to supply very limited information concerning minor events, and a full adverse event form would be inappropriate. A delay until the main record card is returned will not be important for minor events. However, important events will need to be assessed individually for causality and, therefore, more detailed information will be required. There are unlikely to be many similar important events in the two drug groups and they will, therefore, not be suitable for statistical comparison. The important events probably need to be notified to the company before the patient finishes the study and will require subsequent follow-up.

(1)   **Minor events**

   (a)   These are symptom(s) only, which do not warrant stopping or reducing the dose of the drug.

   (b)   No clinical diagnosis has been made.

   (c)   Minimally abnormal laboratory investigations, i.e. insufficient to warrant stopping the drug.

These should be recorded in the record card "clinical notes" or on the laboratory investigation sheet, and the date of onset, duration, frequency, severity (mild, moderate or severe) and outcome should be noted. These will be assessed when the record card is returned to the company. The clinician must be encouraged to give full descriptions of minor events - a single word is not sufficient (see appendix page 231).

(2)   **Important events**

   (a)   All cases which warrant stopping the drug.

   (b)   All cases where a clinical diagnosis has been made.

   (c)   All cases where there are symptoms plus either abnormal physical findings or relevant abnormal laboratory results.

These should be recorded on the adverse event form (page 232), which should be torn out and despatched immediately to the trial sponsor. These cases will be followed up by the company. The latter must be emphasised because otherwise the clinician may delay sending the form until he has more information and there is always a difficulty in deciding whether to notify a possible ADR as soon as the possibility arises or wait until all the data is available and thus establish a causal relationship[140,141]. The follow-up may need to be repeated on several occasions if the results of dechallenge and rechallenge are to be collected. In many studies the single criterion of "warranting the stopping of the drug" can be used to decide between minor and major events.

SPECIAL ADVERSE DRUG REACTION SEARCH

The search for a particular adverse drug reaction which might be foreseen because of:

(1)   Historic reasons – previous similar compounds have been associated with a specific adverse drug reaction, i.e. practolol and a subsequent beta-adrenoceptor antagonist.

(2)   Toxicological reasons – animal studies have identified an area of possible danger.

(3)   Pharmacological reasons – the pharmacology of the drug predicts specific adverse drug reactions : Type A reactions.

(4)   Clinical reasons – adverse drug reactions have occurred in Phase 1 or early Phase 2 studies and are, therefore, foreseen in subsequent studies.

Although it is possible to consider the problems of the non-specific ADR search in clinical trials in general terms, the search for a special ADR based on prior information must be tailored according to the known facts: the drug, the disease it will be used for, the possible duration of treatment and investigational techniques available.

The special studies may be either:

(1)   In special sub-groups of patients with other diseases (see page 69). It is not usually possible to examine the effect of the drug on the complications of the additional illness or in the more severe cases, and this sometimes remains a gap in the knowledge of the drug until spontaneous reporting in the postmarketing period identifies the problem.

(2)   In patients with the target disease only but in whom special investigations are arranged to measure any effect the drug might have on a particular organ or function. This is a difficult area since

the additional investigations are not really in these patients' interest and, if they entail additional clinic visits or unpleasant investigations, are unlikely to be successful. Although all the patients' additional expenses will be refunded, they may need additional incentives. The special investigations usually involve a different discipline to that of the clinical trialist and sometimes a different hospital, all of which adds to the difficulties.

Historical reasons

Literature searches on the ADR of standard therapies will pinpoint important relevant areas. Protocol exclusions frequently reduce the number of patients who might be susceptible to ADR. For each protocol exclusion the decision should be made either to examine the exclusion in a special study before marketing or to make it a contra-indication in the data sheet. The publicity given to the benoxaprofen ADR should ensure that in future differences in drug handling by subsets of patients, i.e. the aged, will be more fully investigated before marketing.

Toxicological reasons

Before the new drug goes into man, discussion with toxicologists will indicate areas which require special attention in man. Differences in absorption, metabolism, distribution and excretion between the animals tested and man should be given special attention.

Pharmacological reasons

Animal toxicology and pharmacology should give advance warning of Type A ADR where objective signs are to be found, but minor ADR with symptoms only will not be found until the drug goes into man.

Clinical reasons

Early in the use of a new drug, either in volunteers or patients, a possible side effect may appear which had not been foreseen for any of the reasons previously mentioned. This possible adverse reaction will then need special attention paid to it in subsequent clinical trials. Two factors need to be considered in searching for an anticipated adverse reaction:

(1)   The expected rarity of the adverse reaction.

(2)   Any predictive factors.

If the anticipated adverse reaction is likely to be common, then it can be sought in clinical trials but, if it is rare, it may need a large scale multicentre study. However, if it is known that certain factors predetermine the patients who will experience the adverse reaction, then special studies can be set up requiring relatively small numbers. "Monitored release studies" or large scale studies in general practice tend to produce the symptoms of adverse reactions rather than diagnoses confirmed by objective data and, as such, do not produce data of the quality one can expect from multicentre hospital studies.

In June 1983 Dr. J. Idanpään-Heikkilä from Finland published the results of a study[169] he undertook whilst on a year's sabbatical leave in the U.S.A. This consisted of a review of safety information obtained in Phase 1, 2, and 3 clinical investigations of sixteen drugs. For Phase 1 studies he concluded that they seemed to uncover certain adverse reactions which are difficult to find in phase 2 and 3 studies and these were:

(1)   ADR that are masked or modified in patients by disease or concomitant medication.

(2)   ADR that are more likely to be induced by higher dosages of the drug.

(3)   ADR that are extensions of the pharmacological action of the drug.

(4)   ADR related to interactions between the drug and common events in daily life to which patients in Phase 2 studies might not be exposed (i.e. alcohol).

Phase 2 studies detect the most frequent adverse reactions and may predict target organ systems for other adverse reactions subsequently discovered in Phase 3 studies. Lack of numbers restricts the possibility of discovering adverse reactions limited to small subgroups and makes it difficult to give accurate incidence figures. He suggested that Phase 2 studies could be extended in time to collect long-term safety data.

Phase 3 studies lasting less than two weeks discover the most frequent and acute adverse reactions and controlled studies demonstrate the actual incidences. Increasing the numbers of patients in these studies from a few hundred to over one thousand does not often detect the rarer adverse reactions (with the exception of antibiotics). It is better to extend the duration of these studies rather than to increase the number of patients since many adverse reactions have long latent periods (three to six months). The author also emphasises the importance of following up dropouts in long-term studies and that the drop-out reduces the number of patients available to suffer adverse reactions with long latent periods. Application of the Life Table Method enables a more accurate estimate of the incidence of these adverse reactions over a period of time. A separate author, Dr. R. T. O'Neill, gives a good account of the Life Table Method in the appendix of the above article.

REPORTING OF CLINICAL TRIALS

The final purpose of a clinical trial is to influence opinion, and the three groups to be influenced are the originating pharmaceutical company, the Regulatory Authorities and the prescribing doctors.

The pharmaceutical company is responsible for the contents of the report on a new drug which is sent to the Regulatory Authority with the request for permission to market the drug. Regulatory Authorities do not make public their assessment of the data submitted to them, but a member of the Finnish Medical Research Council was given permission to study the information submitted to the Finnish and Swedish drug licensing authorities on psychotropic drugs during the period 1950-1977. He commented that much of the information on adverse effects was of poor quality for two reasons: the reports did not say how the adverse effects were defined or determined, and the incidence of adverse effects was either not calculated nor was it related to the efficacy of the drug. The unpublished reports contained more information on adverse effects than the published reports[170].

The results of clinical trials are brought to the prescribing doctor's attention either via the pharmaceutical company's advertising literature or via the publication of the clinical trial results. The former cannot claim objectivity and the latter rarely have sufficient information on ADR[171,172]. A survey of 23 papers published by a reputable medical journal found that 65% of the papers could not be relied upon for specificity, 52% may have been insensitive in their methodology, 88% did not quantify the symptoms observed, 95% failed to characterise susceptible patients and 52% contained no information on dosage in affected patients[167]. Similar criticisms have been made concerning the French medical press[172].

Several checklists have been published for the assessment of clinical trial reports. The checklist used by Information Scientists[173] did not mention ADR, the most relevant questions being "Subjective measurements used to assess effect" and "Objective measurements used to assess effect". In a series of three articles aimed at hospital pharmacists in 1973 entitled "Good and bad clinical trials: a checklist" the author fails to mention ADR[174]. In a communication to the British Pharmacological Society in April 1970 there was a checklist for assessing a therapeutic trial report, also without any mention of ADR[175].

REPORTING OF ADVERSE REACTIONS

Case reports published in the medical journals can be of immense value in warning the prescribers of a new adverse reaction. The problem of erroneous adverse reaction reports could, it has been suggested, be prevented if the reports were first cleared by the Committee on Safety of Medicines[176]. This suggestion was made six years ago but the problem still remains.

A team from a pharmaceutical company reviewed 5,737 articles[177] from 80 countries published between 1972 and 1979 and found that only 61% of these articles included information on the number of patients treated and the number of adverse reactions. In only 55% could the incidence of a particular reaction be calculated.

An analysis[178] of the outcome of 47 anecdotal reports of new adverse reactions published in four major medical journals in 1963 were followed up 18 years later. Fourteen of the 47 reports were considered unlikely to be false positives because they were immediate reactions, local reactions or known reactions caused by a different mode of administration or a brand previously thought or claimed to be safe. The validity of the 33 remaining reports was established in 14 cases, leaving 19 reports needing to be confirmed, but after 18 years twelve of these have still not been confirmed! The fact that of 19 reports which lacked valid evidence at the time of publication 12 remain unconfirmed led the author to suggest that certain criteria should be used to assess the original report's validity. The following criteria should be considered:

(a)   data from rechallenge

(b)   a pharmacological basis for the adverse reaction

(c)   immediate acute adverse reaction

(d)   local reactions at the site of administration

(e)   a first report of reaction with a new route previously recognised with another method of administration

(f)   the repeated occurrence of rare events

This is a further "algorithm" for the assessment of an adverse event. The Bordeaux Pharmacovigilance team have used their own algorithm for a similar purpose[179]. The use of an algorithm may reduce the number of false positive adverse reaction reports appearing in the press but they might also suppress a true adverse reaction report, since they can only reflect the opinion of the assessor.

The readers of articles concerning adverse reaction reports would be best served if the editor submitted the letter to an independent expert and to the pharmaceutical company before publication. The latter would be requested to add comment, if they wished, but it should be confined to comments on the pharmacology of the drug and providing information on the likely incidence of the reaction. This would be published as a footnote to the report. Any other comment by the pharmaceutical company could be submitted for subsequent publication, similar to the present practice.

Guidance for the prescribing doctor, provided by the pharmaceutical companies, is very limited in the field of adverse reactions. Data sheets frequently minimise the adverse effects and do not give the prescriber much help in identifying the patients at risk or advice on dealing with them[180]. A subsidiary document is required, giving details of the adverse reaction profile (see page 17). The medical requirements are frequently in conflict with the commercial demands in the area of information for the prescriber.

CONCLUSIONS

The clinical trial programme for a new drug, as far as adverse reactions are concerned, needs to be based on the known problems found with similar drugs and the results of investigations in animals. The results of the studies in volunteers need to be assessed carefully for potential adverse reactions and then interpreted with previous findings from the animal studies.

Each clinical trial will contribute information concerning the adverse reaction profile of the drug and each protocol should be examined carefully in order to make the most of the drug exposure. The overall trial plan must be balanced such that questionnaires and checklists are used at the right stage with sufficient numbers of patients in order to have a reasonable chance to distinguish between the active drug and its control. The early clinical trials will, whenever possible, try to distinguish the adverse reactions of the new drug from those of placebo-treated patients, whilst later clinical trials will concentrate on comparisons with its potential competitors. Certain of the clinical trials will be allotted to the task of monitoring for specific adverse reactions.

All clinical trial records need to be viewed by intelligent eyes before being put on computer if the opportunity to respond to a potential problem is not to be missed. All patients in clinical trials should be asked at each visit a standard open question and given the opportunity to reply. Adverse symptoms should be followed up by clinical examination and/or investigations to search for objective confirmations. In those cases where the drug is withdrawn, the results of the dechallenge should be observed, preferably without addition of other treatment either substitution for the original drug or for treatment of the adverse reactions, repeating any investigations found to be abnormal at the time of the event.

Uncontrolled studies prior to marketing should be restricted and should be documented and monitored as closely as the normal clinical trials.

5
Postmarketing Surveillance (PMS)

DEFINITION

The term postmarketing surveillance should convey the meaning that the use of a drug after marketing is surveyed both for efficacy and safety; however, as the term is currently used, the emphasis is on safety rather than efficacy. One of the reasons for the lack of emphasis on efficacy has been the fact that the originating pharmaceutical company will organise the necessary studies to demonstrate the efficacy of their products.

The prescribing physician needs to know both about efficacy and safety of a new drug, but not so much in absolute terms but in comparison to previous standard treatments. Few (if any) clinical trials comparing a new drug with the previous standard treatment have sufficient numbers of patients to differentiate between, say, a success rate of the standard drug at 70% and a new drug success rate of 72% with a 95% probability of finding this difference. The reason is that, on the whole, the clinician is not concerned about a 2% difference in efficacy. The lack of efficacy of a drug is usually obvious fairly early on in the course of an illness and a change to an alternative treatment will frequently deal successfully with those two unfortunate patients in every hundred.

However, as mentioned earlier (page 4) with safety, we are dealing with a different order of magnitude of event. The clinician is very concerned about the risk of agranulocytosis with chloramphenicol with an incidence of approximately 1 in 30,000 when compared with any other antibiotic having lesser risk[178]. It is, therefore, right that the pharmaceutical companies should concern themselves with demonstrating the efficacy and safety of their products whilst external agencies concern themselves solely with the safety of these products. Most of the company originated PMS schemes mentioned later in this chapter have concerned themselves both with efficacy and safety, whilst most of the non-company originated schemes are concerned with safety.

One of the differences in these separate approaches to PMS is financial. Efficacy requires, nearly always, objective measurement of changes in every patient by a doctor and this is very expensive compared with the recording of the hopefully rare ADR in the occasional patient. Patient for patient, efficacy is more expensive than ADR reporting. On the other hand, absolute safety is unobtainable[179] and the nearer to absolute safety are the demands of the general population, the more expensive will be the necessary studies. For these reasons the aims of PMS are dealt with only from the ADR point of view, and the different types of PMS are divided into those originating from, and organised by, the pharmaceutical company - in-company schemes - and those originating from, and/or organised by, agencies outside the pharmaceutical companies - the ex-company schemes.

THE PROBLEMS OF PMS

The pre-marketing clinical trial programme will not have covered all the necessary scientific studies which will eventually be required and these will continue to be organised by the research company. Some of the serious ADR subsequently discovered may have been hinted at during the original pre-marketing clinical trials and further studies in these areas will be necessary after marketing. The type of drug and whether it is intended for a single short course or chronic administration will be reflected in the PMS study. All these requirements will be crystallised in the aims of the PMS scheme.

Many different types of studies have been used in PMS and different aims have required different methods for their attainment. Although many pharmaceutical companies have undertaken large-scale uncontrolled post-marketing studies to confirm the efficacy and safety of their products, few have been published with sufficient detail and criticism to further our knowledge of the methodology of this type of study.

AIMS

Political

There are a number of politicians who concern themselves with the pharmaceutical industry and the safety of its products and, similarly, part of the media is interested in the subject and quick to publish details of possible dangerous drug reactions[181]. These two sources reflect the concern of the general public as to the safety of drugs. However, the responses to possible dangers have not always been balanced and have had serious repercussions both on the pharmaceutical industry and the health of the country, e.g. Debendox[25] and pertussis vaccine[183]. These reactions could influence governmental decisions to the detriment of patients[184].

Figure 4 – The aims of PMS

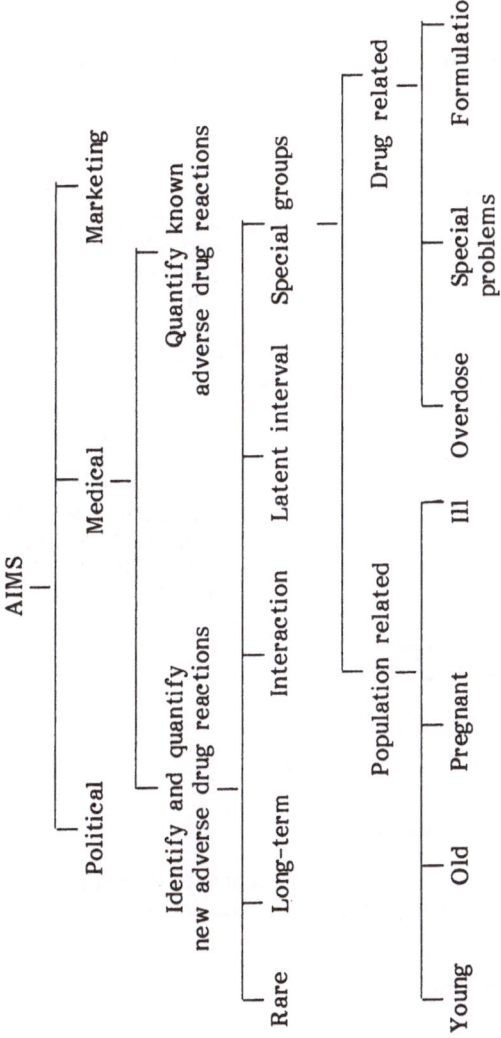

Marketing

Any clinical study which introduces a new drug to a doctor and his patients has a marketing advantage and this may influence the PMS undertaken by the pharmaceutical industry. There will not be much enthusiasm within the industry for an extensive study which requires an equally large control group on another company's drug. All large-scale postmarketing studies organised by pharmaceutical companies must be examined closely to determine to what extent they will influence the prescribing pattern of the new drug.

Medical

ADR with an incidence of 1 in 100 will usually be identified in pre-marketing studies[185] (see **page 10**). The commonest of these will probably be isolated symptoms, i.e. fatigue, nausea, and 90% of ADR will probably appear during the first four days of drug treatment[186]. If one of the aims is to quantify known common ADR, enquiry must be concentrated during that period. It is often not possible to distinguish those symptoms which would have occurred without any treatment, those which would have occurred with a placebo and those caused by the active drug, unless a control is used - either placebo (if the absolute incidence is needed) or against a standard therapy (if a relative incidence is required). A decision to quantify ADR must be made consciously and the best means chosen. It may not be wise to include it as an aim in an uncontrolled study, since the initial enthusiasm for reporting will coincide with the period with the maximum ADR. We will presume that the main medical aim is to identify and quantify, where possible, those ADR not known at the time of marketing and they will be considered under the following headings:

(1)　Rare adverse drug reactions
(2)　Delayed adverse drug reactions
(3)　Interactions
(4)　Latent interval adverse drug reactions
(5)　Special groups

(1)　**Rare adverse drug reactions**

These are considered under the separate headings of specific and non-specific (simulating disease or causing increased incidence of a disease).

Specific adverse drug reactions

Three decisions must be made:-

(1)　What incidence of specific adverse drug reactions do we wish to discover?

(2)   How certain do we wish to be of finding it, i.e. what power is required?

(3)   How many cases do we need in order to establish it as a known reaction?

Non–specific adverse drug reactions

In theory four decisions need to be made:-

(1)   What increase in incidence over and above the natural background incidence do we wish to discover?

(2)   What kind of incidence rate does the naturally occurring disease have?

(3)   What statistical significance should we demand?

(4)   How certain do we wish to be of finding it, i.e. what power?

The discussion of the factors involved in these decisions is in Chapter 1. In practice we do not know which, if any, of the infinite number of naturally occurring diseases the ADR may mimic or simulate and, since that is not known, we cannot say what increase is clinically relevant nor can we know what power we might demand. The aims will vary with the indications for the drug and its intended market. None of the company-organised monitored release schemes has stated an aim in statistical terms with the exception of the U.S.A. Cimetidine Scheme[187] which referred to "specific" ADR rather than non-specific ADR. The aims of a company scheme are more likely to be tailored to what the company can afford in time, staff and money. However, it would be more logical to make an aim in terms of identifying either one or a few cases of a "specific" ADR with a specified incidence and then from the number of patients required to reach this aim calculate what percentage increase in a target disease (e.g. coronary thrombosis) this would identify.

(2)   Long-term adverse drug reactions

How long should a drug study last if it is to detect long-term ADR? There is no upper limit. All long-term studies are plagued with drop-outs and in the United Kingdom arrangements should be made with the N.H.S. (National Health Service) to follow patients once they have left their own practitionr or the district, since 11.3% of patients move annually and over a five-year period 33.4% will move (U.K. Census 1971). The annual rate of changing a practitioner is 9% to 10%[188]. It is, therefore, essential to know the N.H.S. number of the patients. Any study of length will be complicated by withdrawals from treatment or, as mentioned above, by lost patients despite rigorous follow-up. The incidence of adverse events at various stages must be related to the number of patients remaining on the drug at these times. The analysis taking this into account is the Life Table Method[169].

(3)   Interactions

Studies in animals or known interactions of similar drugs may alert one to the need to do specific clinical trials on drug interactions. They may also be discovered by retrospective case-control studies on adverse drug reactions brought to light during PMS schemes.

(4)   Latent interval

The relationship between vaginal adenocarcinoma in young women and the prior intake of diethyl stilboestrol by 7 out of 8 of their mothers during their pregnancy established the problem of the long latent interval in drug monitoring[17]. Case-control studies on unusual clinical entities will probably be the means of discovering any similar problems.

(5)   Special groups

Depending on the range of studies undertaken before marketing, there may be a need to extend surveillance to particular groups of patients either because of population characteristics or drug characteristics.

Population-related characteristics

The pre-marketing clinical trials are usually restricted to a well defined population. There will be little experience as to ADR occurring in the elderly, the young, the pregnant, patients ill with other diseases, or races other than caucasian. This may be tackled once the drug is marketed, either by specific studies or by following a large cohort of patients treated in general practice.

Drug-related characteristics

Animal studies or previous problems with drugs of the same group may indicate areas where special surveillance is needed.

Different formulations of a drug can cause different ADR due to pharmacokinetic differences. These may require special studies. If ADR are dose-related, problems of overdosage may not be seen until the drug is marketed. The whole area of self-poisoning is an important aspect of PMS and provision needs to be made for it.

Figure 5 : Different types of P.M.S. (ex-company)

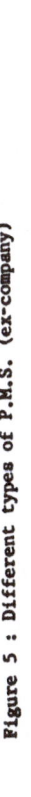

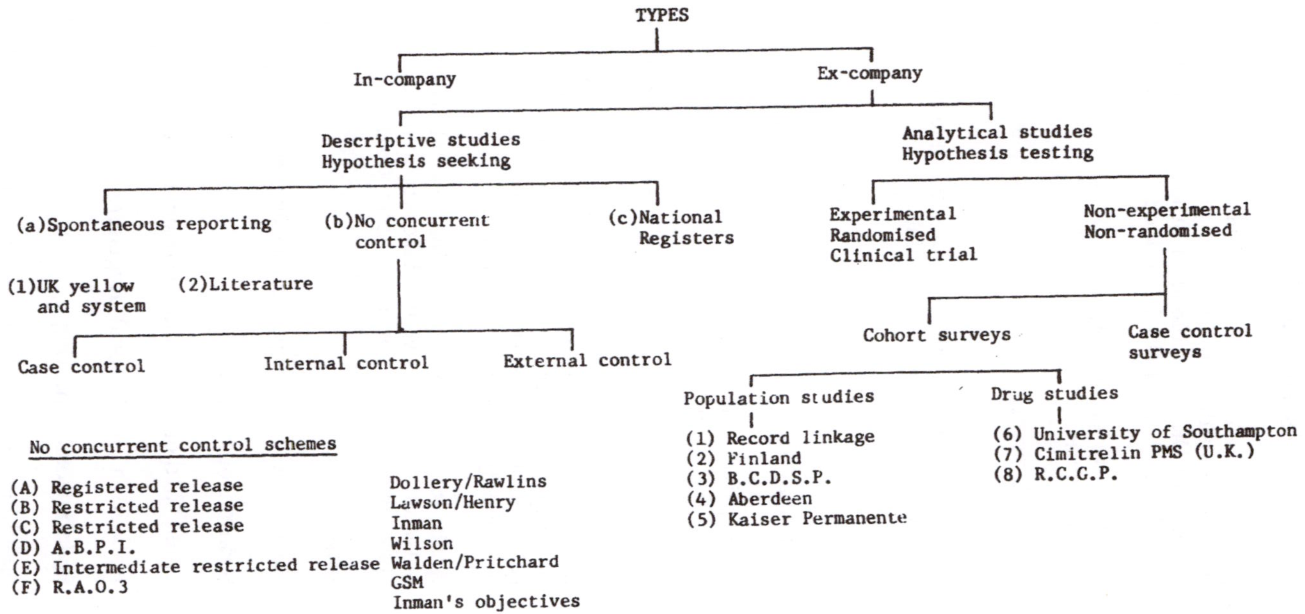

TYPES

In-company — Ex-company

(a) Spontaneous reporting
(1) UK yellow and system
(2) Literature

Case control — Internal control — External control

Descriptive studies Hypothesis seeking
(b) No concurrent control
(c) National Registers

Analytical studies Hypothesis testing

Experimental Randomised Clinical trial — Non-experimental Non-randomised

Cohort surveys — Case control surveys

Population studies — Drug studies

Population studies:
(1) Record linkage
(2) Finland
(3) B.C.D.S.P.
(4) Aberdeen
(5) Kaiser Permanente

Drug studies:
(6) University of Southampton
(7) Cimitrelin PMS (U.K.)
(8) R.C.G.P.

No concurrent control schemes

(A) Registered release — Dollery/Rawlins
(B) Restricted release — Lawson/Henry
(C) Restricted release — Inman
(D) A.B.P.I. — Wilson
(E) Intermediate restricted release — Walden/Pritchard
(F) R.A.O.3 — GSM
Inman's objectives

DIFFERENT TYPES OF PMS

Having decided on the medical aims of PMS with a new drug, it is necessary to consider the various possible types of studies available in order to choose the right blend of studies most suited to the drug. For the purposes of this book PMS is divided into two main parts:

(1)   The PMS undertaken without or with only minimal involvement of the pharmaceutical company.

(2)   The PMS programme that has been undertaken by a pharmaceutical company.

More emphasis will be placed on the industry-based PMS but the non-industry involvement will be outlined.

Ex-company

The division of the main types of PMS into

(1)   descriptive studies, and
(2)   analytical studies

is based on whether or not one is seeking or testing a hypothesis.

(1)   Descriptive studies describe events related to drug efficacy and adverse drug reactions in various populations and, therefore, may associate an event with a drug but do not establish a causal relationship. Since they do not have a concurrent control group, they are mainly hypothesis seeking.

(2)   Analytical studies determine causal relationships or associations between drug and event. Since they have a concurrent control group they can be used for hypothesis testing.

Descriptive Studies

There are three main types of descriptive study:

(a)   Spontaneous reporting

(b)   Those without a randomised concurrent control group

(c)   Inspection of National Registers

(a)   **Spontaneous reporting**

Spontaneous reporting covers reporting in the literature as well as the voluntary reporting system (yellow cards) in the U.K.

1.   **U.K. "Yellow Card" System**

This is voluntary in the U.K. but a similar system is mandatory in Sweden. Enforcement in Sweden produced a 25% increase in reporting[190,191]. The system in the U.K. has had numerous successes:

(1) .   Halothane - jaundice[192,198]

(2)   Oestrogens and thrombo-embolism[193,194]

(3)   Protriptyline - photosensitivity[8]

(4)   Nalidixic acid - CNS effects[195]

(5)   Ibufenac and liver damage[196]

(6)   Mianserin-induced arthropathy[197]

(7)   Amiodarone-induced hepatitis[197]

(8)   Piroxicam-induced congestive cardiac failure[197]

(9)   Methyldopa and hepatitis[198]

(10)   Metoclopramide and extrapyramidal side effects[198]

but it has had its failures:

(1)   Practolol oculomucocutaneous syndrome[198]

(2)   Incorrect identification of erythromycin estolate as being a more important cause of jaundice than other esters[199].

Advantages

(a)   Confidential

(b)   Large number of exposed patients

(c)   The clustering of reports around a drug can provide early warning of an unsuspected effect. Comparison of the pattern of ADR produced by chemically similar drugs can identify relative increases in incidence of ADR. International co-operation increases the size of the pool of patients since 23 countries report their ADR to the W.H.O. international project on drug monitoring.

Disadvantages

(a)   Gross under-reporting (estimated reporting only 1 to 10%)[75].

(b)   Biased reporting favouring previously reported ADR

(c)   No denominator and, therefore, no incidence rates.

(d)   It cannot provide evidence of a causal relationship between a drug and the ADR

(e)   The amount of information which can be given to the pharmaceutical companies is very limited.

Overall comment

It is and will remain an essential part of PMS, especially for comparing one product with other members of the same group. Although there is believed to be gross under-reporting in the U.K. (10,179 reports in 1980) and in Sweden[200], it is considerably better than in France and West Germany with 6,000 reports per annum and 2,500 reports per annum respectively – both countries with similar total populations[201]. It would probably be improved if all pharmaceutical representatives stimulated prescribing doctors to report ADR, as described on page 112. The First Report of the Working Party on Adverse Reactions (see page 190) recommends certain steps to increase spontaneous reporting.

2.   **Literature**

Individual astute clinicians will always be the most likely discoverers of very rare ADR. Their successes are many:

(1)   amino fumarate – primary pulmonary hypertension[202].

(2)   phenylbutazone – leucopenia[203].

(3)   methyldopa – haemolytic anaemia[204].

(4)   chloramphenicol – aplastic anaemia[205].

(5)   practolol – oculomucocutaneous syndrome[206].

Disadvantages

(a)   Physicians may delay reporting to the C.S.M. in order to write up their own series of cases.

(b)   It cannot give incidence rates of adverse reactions.

Advantages

(a)   Has been the most prolific source for the discovery of very rare adverse drug reactions.

(b)   Often well documented.

(c)   An initial report may stimulate other doctors to describe their own experience – the so-called "halo" or "boule de neige" effect – and may, therefore, confirm or dispute what was originally a rather doubtful case.

Overall

It will continue to be the most important source of reports of serious ADR. The high success rate (75%) of this source suggests that only "probable" reports are published[178].

The criteria used by journals vary considerably in the proof they demand before publication of a possible ADR. When ADR mentioned in letters to the British Medical Journal for the year 1963 were followed up in 1980, 25% were found to be unconfirmed[178]. Publication of the association of a drug with an adverse effect with no suggestion of its causal relationship such that any "possible" relationships are included could improve the results without causing unnecessary alarm.

(b) **Schemes with no randomised concurrent control group**

Although these schemes (both in-company and ex-company) are mainly descriptive and hypothesis seeking, there are three ways in which they can test hypotheses:-

(1) Case control studies

(2) External control studies

(3) Internal control studies

1. **Case control studies**

If the trial drug (A) is suspected of interacting with another drug (B) to produce an adverse event, the records of patients with the event are examined to find the number of patients who received and did not receive drug B. These numbers are then related to the total number of patients receiving drug A and drug B respectively. A Chi-squared test will show whether there is a significant difference between the proportion of those patients taking drug B and drug A and having the event and those taking drug A alone and having the event. The possibility of drug B by itself causing the event then has to be excluded by inspection of the records.

2. **External control studies**

The external control may be a historic control, i.e. certain side effects may be less when patients are transferred to a new drug than whilst they were on their previous treatment. However, with external controls there are often confounding factors. One might be tempted to draw the conclusion that a new drug had less side effects than other previous drugs for the same indication but, of course, those patients on the previous drugs who had no side effects had less of a chance of being given the new drug. Another external control group often used is the Registrar General's figures. Where independent agencies survey drug cohorts, the results of a previous cohort study of a similar drug may act as a control group, provided the survey methods are comparable.

3.   **Internal control studies**

These may be of two types:

(1)   in patients

(2)   between patients.

(i)   **In patients**

This is a comparison of the adverse events suffered by the patient during the period before or after taking the drug compared with the period whilst on the drug. Both are open to considerable bias. The adverse events prior to the drug will be complicated by the disease requiring treatment and frequently previous therapy. The period after the drug may conceal delayed ADR due to the drug. There will be an inherent bias towards reporting adverse events during treatment against reporting them after treatment. A good method for dealing with this has been described by Dr. Inman in P.E.M. (see page 105).

(ii)   **Between patients**

It is often useful to know what factors might predict certain ADR. The results of patients with the factor are compared with those without that factor, and the result is a retrospective cohort study. The comparison between the incidence of adverse events in the two groups of patients can often help characterise the event, i.e. male:female; over 65 years:under 65 years, etc.

A   **Registered release**[207]

Put forward by Dollery and Rawlins in 1977:

Features

(i)   No free sales until a registered quota has been completed and, therefore, there would be a delay in the normal marketing of the drug.

(ii)   Doctors would fill in a 4-part no-carbon-required form and would require payment.

(iii)   Follow-up both to patient and doctor once a year for five years.

(iv)   All deaths in monitored group logged by Office of Population and Census Survey.

(v)   Run by registering agency.

(vi)   Recruitment by pharmaceutical representatives.

(vii)   Not yet tried in practice, although many features were incorporated in the PMS scheme for atenolol.

Disadvantages

(a)   Expensive.

(b)   It will reduce sales.

(c)   It will delay general use of the drug.

(d)   There would not be a control group for questionnaires.

(e)   The use of sales representatives may distort the distribution of monitoring doctors.

(f)   It has been suggested that, if the patient answers a questionnaire, this will upset the normal doctor-patient relationship.

(g)   It might require new legislation to restrict prescribing to monitoring doctors.

(h)   The knowledge that the drug is being monitored will alter prescribing habits.

Advantages

(a)   It would replace "promotional" schemes organised and run by pharmaceutical companies.

(b)   It is the only scheme to collect information from patients.

This was the initial scheme and other people have improved on it, but it established some of the principles.

B   ## Restricted or monitored release[208]

Lawson and Henry put this forward in March 1977.

Features

(i)   Drug prescriptions would be collected by pharmacists.

(ii)   Follow-up by G.P. for hospital attendances and death.

(iii)   Fee to pharmacists but not to G.P.

(iv)   Independent registration body to organise the system.

Disadvantages

(a)   May not represent a truly random selection of the population at risk.

(b)   The failure to collect G.P. diagnoses and non-hospital events may result in missing an adverse reaction.

Advantages

(a)   Could be localised to a region.

(b)   Less expensive - would not change prescribing habits.

Overall comment

Lawson has reported on a similar modified system which will be described further   (page 106).   The co-operation by G.P.s and pharmacists has been good.

C   **Recorded release**[209]

This was put forward by Inman (June 1977)

Features

(i)   Would require special FP10 prescription forms.

(ii)   All patients to be followed up.

Disadvantages

(a)   Special form would probably distort prescribing habits.

(b)   Would collect all adverse events and "reasons for any con-sultation".

Advantages

(a)   Rapid recruitment likely.

(b)   Would involve both hospital doctors and G.P.s

Overall comment

Has all the disadvantages of major G.P. involvement, i.e. cost, and was subsequently revised by Dr. Inman.

D   **Pharmaceutical Industry scheme**

Put forward in October 1977 by Wilson[210].

Features

(i)   Similar to above scheme but the Prescription Pricing Authority (P.P.A.) would collect prescriptions.

(ii)   Independent agency to organise it.

(iii) Questionnaire to doctors similar to the above scheme.

Disadvantages

P.P.A. may not be as adept at reading the doctor's prescriptions as local pharmacists.

Advantages

(a)   Avoids the use of pharmacists and, therefore, reduces the cost and possible bias.

(b) Will not affect prescribing practice.

Overall comment

A possible improvement on the monitored release.

E   **Intermediate restricted release**

This was put forward by Walden and Pritchard[211]

Features

(i)   Half-way between clinical trials and monitored release.

(ii)   Would entail specially modified G.P. prescription forms.

(iii) Would involve a central agency and the pharmaceutical company concerned.

(iv)   Would use a simple report form for results of efficacy and safety.

(v)   Only special doctors allowed to prescribe and all patients to be monitored.

Disadvantages

(a)   Special prescription used by special doctors would disturb the normal prescribing pattern.

(b)   Request for evidence of efficacy would increase the costs.

(c)   Involvement of pharmaceutical company would be controversial.

Advantages

(a)   Reduction of number of patients monitored would mean fewer patients at risk.

(b)   Would monitor hospital doctors as well as G.P.s

F   **Retrospective Assessment of Drug Safety (R.A.D.S.)**

R.A.D.S. was put foward by the C.S.M.[212]

Features

(i)   Retrospective and, therefore, the drug need not be declared publicly.

(ii)   Would record clinical events.

(iii)   Follow-up of 10,000 of the patients receiving the drug from the first 100,000 prescriptions.

(iv)   Prescriptions picked up by P.P.A.

(v)   Turned down by Government because of costs.

Disadvantages

G.P.s might have a bias in their reporting, choosing to report on those with few adverse events and not those with many.

Advantages

(a)   No effect on prescribing habits.

(b)   Little medico-legal risk.   Avoidance of bias of prospective study.

Overall comment

Possibly expensive.   The increased detail demanded from the prescribing doctor could make compliance a problem.

Inman's objectives

The pros and cons of the various systems have been discussed in the medical press[213-217] without coming out in favour of any one scheme. The problem of all the systems mentioned is that there are no concurrent controls and, therefore, the only external controls possible would be historical controls, i.e. using previous drugs that have gone through the scheme as controls for the next. Inman has put forward a series of objectives for his   recorded   release scheme[217].

1.   It should measure the incidence of adverse events of various kinds among patients exposed to the test drug.

2.   Adverse events should be ascertained and recorded, whether or not the observer believes them to be drug-related.

3.   All patients receiving the new drug should be monitored until sufficient time has elapsed or numbers accumulated for non-negligible risks to be assessed.

4.   The system should include arrangements for long-term follow-up.

5.   It should ensure rapid communication among those who have observed the adversities, the monitoring organisation, and the drug's manufacturer.

6.   There should be no limitation of a doctor's freedom to prescribe the drug or the patient's right to derive benefit from it.

7.   Medico-legal risks should be minimised.

8.   The arrangements must be standardised so that the results of studying the different drugs may be compared.

9.   As far as possible, normal marketing conditions should be simulated.

10.   Development time (the time from the first patient taking the drug in clinical trials to the time it is available to all patients in the U.K.) should not be increased.

11. The arrangements for recording drug exposures or patient adversities must be simple.

12. Costs should be kept low.

DISCUSSION

The use of a patient questionnaire in a PMS scheme without a control group is likely to cause some problems. Firstly, patients are likely to record symptoms rather than diagnoses and these by themselves are difficult to interpret. Secondly, questionnaires are likely to produce anxiety in some patients and may disturb the doctor-patient relationship and, in order to avoid this, the doctor might exclude certain types of patients.

Both recorded release (Inman) and R.A.D.S. require the collection by the doctor of "the reasons for any consultation" without specifying that it is the diagnosis that should be recorded, and this would probably result in the collection of symptoms. The recording of symptoms is not appropriate to a long-term PMS scheme for the reasons mentioned in Chapter 2, page 26.

It would be important for the central organising agency to have continuing experience of monitoring so that continued employment of the staff could be assured and experience gained. This would also enable the comparison with previous drugs if historic controls were required. In order to assure the agency continuous work, the number of agencies for the U.K. would need to be limited to two or three and would preclude the pharmaceutical companies from acting as agencies. If the results of PMS were to be accepted by foreign regulatory authorities, it would be necessary for the central agency to be seen to be independent of the pharmaceutical industry.

The three main advantages that PMS has over pre-marketing studies are:

(1) There is a much larger pool of patients.

(2) The drug is prescribed by all sorts of doctors.

(3) The drug is prescribed for all sorts of patients.

If any of these three advantages is lost, then the results cannot be extrapolated to the whole population. It is, therefore, important that prescribing should not be limited to a particular kind of doctor. For this same reason the prescribing doctor should not know that the drug will be the subject of monitoring, lest it alter his prescribing habits. Retrospective studies have the advantage that the doctor need not be concerned with the monitoring until the required period has elapsed and, therefore, his prescribing will not be affected. However, for the same reason he is unlikely to pay sufficient attention to any adverse event and it is likely to be under-investigated compared with the same event in a prospective study.

The Prescription Pricing Authority (P.P.A.) has had experience of collecting normal prescriptions for a survey[216] and this would not necessitate special forms (FP10).

All descriptive schemes have, by definition, no concurrent control group and, therefore, can only propose hypotheses whilst analytical studies with a concurrent control group can test hypotheses. Historical or retrospective controls are not nearly as satisfactory as concurrent controls. The addition of a control group to the Henry/Lawson scheme is represented by the PMS of cimetidine in the U.K. by Smith Kline & French with which Lawson has been associated, and the addition of a control group to R.A.D.S. is represented by the University of Southampton Prescription Event Monitoring. The two schemes will be discussed on pages 105 and 106.

CONCLUSIONS

The criteria for an ideal PMS scheme for the detection of ADR with a frequency greater than 1 in 1,000 are the twelve objectives put forward by Inman with the addition of a further two:

(1)   A concurrent control group should be incorporated (as in Dr. Inman's scheme), although patients could not be randomly allocated to the trial or control drug.

(2)   The number of organising agencies in the U.K. should probably be not more than three.

DESCRIPTIVE STUDIES

National Registers

In the U.K. linkage of Office of Population Censuses & Surveys (O.P.C.S.) data with National Health Service Register Number in the National Cancer Registry could identify delayed carcinogenic effects. Unfortunately, death certificates are often inaccurate[76,77,219]. The Registrar General's figures for deaths, the O.P.C.S. register of congenital abnormalities and the national register of hospital admissions have proved valuable in providing hypotheses. The successes from this system have been: the oral contraceptive – pulmonary thromboembolism study[193,194], and children's asthma mortality – pressurised aerosol study[9]. Both studies also involved the C.S.M.'s voluntary reporting system.

P.M.S. : Table 19

	Ex-company. No con control group schemes	Dollery & Rawlins	Lawson & Henry	Inman*	A.B.P.I.	R.A.D.S.	Walden & Pritchard
Action required by	Patient	X		?			
	G.P.	X	X	X	X	X	X
	Hospital doctor			X			X
	Pharmacist		X				
	P.P.A.			X	X	X	
	C.S.M.					X	
	Reps.	X					
Organiser	Ph. Co.	?	?				X
	C.S.M.	?	?			X	
	R.C.G.P.	?	?	?			
	A.B.P.I.		?	?			
	Pharm. Soc.		?	?			
	Not stated			X			X
Information from doctor	Symptoms			X		X	?
	G.P. diagnosis	X		X	X	X	?
	Hospital diagnosis	X	X	X	X	X	?
	Hospital referrals	X					?
	Died		X	X	X	X	?
	Efficacy						X
Prescribing freedom	Restricted	X		X			X
	Not restricted		X		X	X	
Documents	4-part N.C.R.	X				.	
	Single form		X				
	FP10 photocopy				X	X	
	Modified FP10			X			X

```
P.P.A.    = Prescription Pricing Authority
A.B.P.I. = Association of British Pharmaceutical Industry
N.C.R.    = No carbon required
FP10      = Standard form for NHS prescriptions
Ph. Co.  = Pharmaceutical company
R.A.D.S. = Retrospective assessment of drug safety
Reps.    = Pharmaceutical company representative
```

* Dr. Inman P.E.M. study uses either a histone control group or a concurrent control group.

In the U.S.A. there are numerous specialised adverse reaction registers:

(1)   Hepatitis
(2)   Eye
(3)   Radio-contrast media
(4)   Tissue (pathology)
(5)   Radio-pharmaceutical

as well as other data sources which can be used in PMS:

(a)   Drug abuse warning network
(b)   Birth defect registry
(c)   National morbidity, mortality data (National Centre for Health Statistics)

ANALYTICAL STUDIES - EXPERIMENTAL AND NON-EXPERIMENTAL

Any of the systems mentioned so far may originate a hypothesis relating to a drug and an ADR.   In order to test this hypothesis one must look to an analytical method.   These are divided into randomised and non-randomised studies and it is the former, where there is a randomised choice of active drug and concurrent control, which forms the basis of all clinical testing - the formal clinical trial.   Since this is the only form of PMS which is relatively free from bias[220], it should be the pharmaceutical industry's main tool.   If we now turn to the non-randomised controlled trial, then it will be obvious that it is open to bias.

There are two types of non-randomised controlled trials:

(1)   Cohort surveys

(2)   Case control surveys.

Cohort Surveys

These may be prospective or retrospective.   In the latter it is necessary to define retrospectively the treatment cohorts one wishes to study and then treat as a prospective cohort study, i.e. Inman's Prescription Event Monitoring.   In the prospective cohort study the cohort or group in which the patient is placed is usually not determined randomly and the doctor chooses the treatment openly with the result that his judgment will be biased as to which treatment a patient will have, either by preconceived notions concerning the drug or the patient's clinical state.   Once a bias is recognised, it can be partially countered by groupings according to known variables.

The cohort studies can also be divided into two groups:

(a)   Where the cohort is chosen by the particular population.

(b)   Where the cohort is chosen by the treatment they are given.

Population Cohort Studies

There have been many of these and five will be selected to represent the whole field.   The fate of the user of a drug is compared with that of the non-user[221].

(1)   Record Linkage in England - Oxford[222] and Tayside[227].

(2)   Record Linkage abroad - Finland[223].

(3)   Hospital in-patient population - Boston Collaborative Drug Survey Programme, U.S.A.   Intensive surveillance[224].

(4)   Hospital in-patient population U.K. - Aberdeen.   Intensive surveillance[225].

(5)   Hospital out-patient population - Kaiser Permanente Drug Monitoring System[226].

1.   <u>Record linkage, Oxford, England</u>[221]

The Oxford Record Linkage Study was begun in 1962.   Records of births, deaths, hospital admissions and obstetric deliveries, general practice prescriptions and general practice records have been linked.   Using this system they were able to identify patients who had received practolol and their case notes were examined for eye complaints and rashes.   Of the 71 patients, 20% had eye complaints during practolol treatment compared with 6% during a comparative period before practolol treatment.   There was a statistically significant difference ($P<0.01$).

<u>Tayside Record Linkage Study</u>[227]

The population involved is now 400,000 and will increase to 1.2 million when the Grampian and Argyll & Clyde Health Boards have the same system.   Each patient has a Community Health Number (C.H. No.). Photocopies of prescriptions are obtained from the Prescription Pricing Division and can be cross-linked to the C.H. No. held by the Area Health Board which is linked to the hospital discharge diagnoses (coded to 9th revision of the I.C.D.) and the O.P.C.S. Classification of Surgical Operations.   Linkage can also be obtained with Maternity and cross-referenced to the children and then to the Child Development Scheme. It is limited to serious ADR, i.e. requiring reference to a hospital, and therefore complements Prescription Event Monitoring and depends on the accuracy of the hospital discharge diagnoses.   Its advantages are that it can continue to monitor indefinitely, should pick up potential teratogens, does not require any third party co-operation, pre-prescription morbidity can be investigated and, since the system was originally installed for another purpose, the additional cost is small. A successful pilot study with cimetidine has been carried out at a cost of just over £12,000 for a 3,800 patient survey.

2.   Record Linkage, Finland[223]

Five health surveillance registers cover Finland and they are all computerised. They are:

(i)   Cancer Register

(ii)   Congenital malformation register

(iii)   Hospital discharge register

(iv)   Drug adverse reaction register

(v)   Register of persons entitled to free drugs

They have used the system successfully for monitoring the incidence of digitalis intoxication and for a case control study on reserpine and breast cancer and for the discovery that clozapine could cause fatal agranulocytosis.

3.   Hospital In-patient Population – Boston Collaborative Drug Survey Programme[224]

This is based on 19 hospitals in six countries. Data is collected from all in-patients by trained nurse monitors or pharmacist monitors. The monitors interview patients, and physicians collect information on all drugs prescribed or discontinued, adverse reactions and discharges, and all of these are computerised. They have presented findings on:

(i)   the epidemiology of digoxin, spironolactone, propranolol, intravenous diazepam and tricyclic antidepressants.

(ii)   association between adverse drug reactions and intravenous ethacrynic acids, penicillins, analgesics and dipyrone.

(iii)   predisposing factors to efficacy or toxicity of heparin, prednisone, diphenylhydantoin, chlordiazepoxide, diazepam, propoxyphene and digoxin.

(iv)   interactions between chloral hydrate and warfarin, ampicillin and allopurinol, and tetracyclines and diuretics.

Advantages

(1)   Causal relationships and incidence rates can be established.

(2)   All relevant data recorded.

Disadvantages

(1)   Only studies a hospital population over a relatively short   period.

(2)   Relatively high cost and a complex organisation.

4.   Hospital In-patient - Aberdeen-Dundee System[225]

This was originally based, in the mid-sixties, on the Aberdeen hospitals alone but has been extended to cover the Dundee hospitals since 1972. Data concerning each patient discharged is collected from the Scottish Hospital Morbidity Return and from the prescribing records, so that patient identification and diagnoses are linked to the drugs prescribed. The system covers some 4,300 beds with a discharge rate of 70,000 per annum.   The system has been used for testing the association between spironolactone and breast cancer (negative), methaqualone and peripheral neuritis (negative) as well as the cardiotoxicity of amitriptyline, psychomimetic effects of pentazocine and dihydrocodeine tartrate, rauwolfia derivatives and breast cancer, L-dopa and direct anti-globin tests.

5.   Hospital Out-patient - Kaiser-Permanente Drug Monitoring System, U.S.A.[226]

Based in San Francisco between 1966 and 1973 and served about 120,000 patients.   All out-patients were monitored.   Probably over 80% of out-patient prescriptions actually filled in were dispensed in the hospital.   All diagnoses and adverse drug reactions were linked.   The primary search was for statistical association between drugs and events with subsequent evaluation to determine the existence of a cause and effect relationship. The system has been used to discover the relationship between oral contraceptives and candida vaginitis, frusemide and gout, tolbutamide and congestive heart failure.   In 1973 F.D.A. support for the Kaiser-Permanente Outpatient Surveillance was withdrawn[228].   A similar Kaiser-Permanente Scheme is operating in Los Angeles.   These are examples of Health Maintenance Organisations (H.M.O.), the biggest of which is Medicaid, a pharmaceutical analysis and surveillance system[229].

In general it is possible to estimate the incidence of side effects in various treatment groups and also to establish the power of the test but obviously they are not as valid scientifically as are controlled randomised trials but probably more so than case-control studies.   In many of the schemes just mentioned it is also possible to conduct case control studies or drug-oriented cohort studies but some schemes have been designed to monitor a single drug.

Drug-oriented Cohort Studies

There are three non-industry drug studies which come under this heading in the U.K.

6.   Prescription Event Monitoring - Drug Surveillance Research Unit, University of Southampton

Established in 1980 by Dr. Inman[39]

Features

(1)   Prescriptions for the drug identified by the Prescription Pricing Authority (P.P.A.), photocopied and passed to the Unit.

(2)   A similar but established drug will be used as a control.   Only patients who are newly prescribed the drugs will be followed.

(3)   A questionnaire will be sent to the doctor after, say, one year, requesting details of new diagnoses and hospital attendances or new events.   The definition used for event includes "any complaint of symptoms that were not present before the treatment was started". The G.P. will not be paid.   Confidentiality will be absolute.

Advantages

(1)   Does not alter prescribing habits.

(2)   Since no medical opinion is requested - no fee will be paid and, therefore, it should be relatively cheap.

(3)   There will be a reasonable control group (unrandomised).

Disadvantages

The bias affecting which patient has the drug under test and which has the control must be identified and dealt with (see page 70).   Since dealing with the bias will probably require asking the G.P. further   questions, the cost may increase.

The inclusion of a request to the G.P. to record new symptoms might produce three problems:

(1)   The G.P. either not complying with the request or demanding a fee for the increased work.   So far, however, there has been no problem and the expected response rate[230] is over 50%.

(2)   Swamping the system with meaningless symptoms.

(3)   If the two groups are compared for symptoms, diagnoses and ADR, the number of possible statistical comparisons will be vast with the

result that, if a significance level of 5% is used, there will be many follow-ups to be done merely because of chance positive results. If this is to be avoided, then the level of significance needs to be altered to 5%/K (where K = the possible number of classes available for analysis). However, this will result in loss of sensitivity[231]. At the moment there is no satisfactory answer to the problem.

(4)   The patients of the doctors not replying (50%) may have a different adverse event incidence than those patients of the doctors replying, i.e. G.P.s with patients with voluminous notes may be less likely to report than G.P.s of those with minimal notes.

The use of adverse reaction profiles in a histogram format will be similar to the systems used by the C.S.M. for monitoring voluntary reported adverse reactions and have already shown up the photosensitivity of benoxaprofen compared with fenbrufen[232].

When Dr. Inman applied his system to ranitidine, instead of using another drug as a control he compared the adverse events occurring during this period on ranitidine with the period after ranitidine treatment. The ratio of adverse events per month on treatment compared with that after treatment was 1.2:1. Plotting of individual adverse events showed the expected scatter of ratios on either side of the mean ratio 1.2:1. Those with ratios of greater than 1.2:1 were potential adverse effects and, therefore, generated hypotheses which then required investigation in a separate hypothesis testing database. A copy of the first report from the Drug Surveillance Research Unit is available from Dr. Inman.

Overall comment

This is the best of all the alternatives at the moment.

7.   Postmarketing surveillance of cimetidine

This has been organised by Lawson et al[233].

Features

(1)   10,000 patients taking cimetidine were followed for 18 months.

(2)   Pharmacists identified prescriptions in three main centres: Portsmouth, Oxford and Glasgow, and the pharmacist was paid a fee, whilst in Nottingham the prescriptions were collected by the Prescription Pricing Authority.

(3)   The G.P. was visited by a monitor three months after the prescription had been given and she identified a control patient from the practitioner's files, matching for sex and age group but not for disease. The practitioner was not paid.

(4)   A further visit took place at 18 months, and all data on hospitali-
       sation, hospital attendance, death or cessation of cimetidine due to
       side effects were obtained.

(5)   The scheme worked well with 90% co-operation from the pharmacists
       and 60% from the doctors[234].

Disadvantages

The fact that the patients were not matched with another patient with a
peptic ulcer meant that the cimetidine group was biased by any problems
associated with peptic diseases.   This was a confounding factor.   An
increase in adverse events in the cimetidine group was identified[235] but
the reason for this is not known.

Advantages

Did not influence prescribing habits. It was relatively cheap. Independent
of the marketing company.

Overall comment

Should be a very close second to Inman's scheme at the University of
Southampton.

8.   The Royal College of General Practice[236]

The College has set up a Medicines Surveillance Organisation and is
recruiting 1,600 general practitioners from the College membership for the
surveillance of a new analgesic, sutoprofen. Each practitioner will monitor
six patients for a period of six months and will report all adverse events.
In addition, both the patient and the doctor will comment on the
effectiveness of the treatment.   The practitioner will be paid £6 per
patient.   The organisation will also monitor a second drug, meptazinol,
which will not be marketed until a substantial amount of data has
accumulated despite the fact that it is already licensed for marketing.
Ten thousand patients will be monitored for a period of fourteen days and
a subset of 2,000 for one year.   Any complaints of side effects will be
noted.   At four weeks all events which have occurred will be collected so
that it will be possible to compare the adverse events during two weeks on
the drug and for two weeks after the drug. The study will be analysed by
the pharmaceutical company.   A report will be written in collaboration
with the director of the R.C.G.P. organisation and the manufacturers.

Disadvantages

(1)   In the pilot study, of the doctors chosen randomly only half recruited
       patients and one third followed them up for one year.

(2)   Probably altered prescribing habits in one third of doctors.

(3)   The only control will be the period immediately after taking the drug so that it will only be a hypothesis seeking study.

These last three agencies have been financed, at least partly, by the pharmaceutical industry.

Case-control surveys

With these one starts with the cases with the possible adverse reaction and then retrospectively chooses the controls without the possible adverse reaction.   To try to prevent bias[237-241], the controls are matched as closely as possible for all factors other than the possible adverse reaction but the problems involved are many.   The two groups are then compared for drug usage. Since collecting the data is retrospective, there is unlikely to be any standardisation.   The patients presenting with the possible adverse reaction may not represent the population at large and the incidence of the possible adverse reaction cannot be determined.   By the nature of case control, it is frequently used by clinicians when faced with unusual diagnoses, i.e. vaginal adenocarcinoma in young women in their twenties is extremely rare so that when Herbst et al[17] saw 8 cases and found that 7 of them had a history of having had diethyl stilboestrol via their mothers during pregnancy, the method used was case-control survey.   This method has the advantage that it is relatively quick and cheap and is most applicable to rare drug-related events but requires the drug to be widely prescribed.

Pharmaceutical companies are rarely involved in these studies since the population with the rare adverse event/disease will not be available to the pharmaceutical company.   However, a prospective international case-control study has been undertaken on behalf of Hoechst A.G.[242] and a case study initiated by I.C.I. on Peyronie's disease[243].

DISCUSSION

The record linkage schemes in Oxford and Finland have a proven record of efficiency.   The Oxford scheme links general practitioner prescriptions and diagnoses with hospital admissions and diagnoses and all deaths for a population of 42,000 but does not deal with hospital prescriptions[222]. Although it is capable of expansion, it cannot cover the whole community due to the cost and workload which would be involved.   The Finnish scheme, linking as it does six different systems, can only monitor registered adverse drug reactions, cancer, congenital malformations, hospital discharges and persons entitled to free drugs, so the emphasis tends to be on hospital rather than general practice.   The system is peculiar to Finland and, although the principles could be applied in the U.K., the U.K. population would probably be more resistant to the storage of so much personal information by the state.   An additional advantage of record linkage is that it can be grafted on to existing data collection systems originally started for management purposes, so keeping the cost down. They are probably the most useful hypothesis testing schemes since the results can be available in a very short time after the hypothesis has been advanced.

Intensive hospital surveillance as in the B.C.D.S.P. and the Aberdeen/Dundee system is expensive and, therefore, must be limited to a few hospitals only but does provide a unique source of ADR data.

The Kaiser-Permanente Drug Monitoring System covered out-patients but had a limited value since in-patient data was not recorded. It was limited in membership to about 120,000 patients in San Francisco and this was probably not representative of the rest of the U.S.A. Since it was based on a private health management organisation, its principles could not so easily apply to the U.K.[227]. Its government financing was withdrawn in 1973 and, therefore, this drug surveillance programme no longer functions[228] but similar projects are functioning at Los Angeles and Puget Sound, Seattle.

The Medicaid System has been adopted by the F.D.A. for drug surveillance of both in- and out-patients and covers approximately 2.5 million patients, including 600,000 children of less than 15 years and 350,000 elderly patients[229].

All the schemes discussed so far are related to populations and, as far as the U.K. is concerned, are unlikely ever to be applied to the whole population. The U.K. contributions to these schemes have shown their worth and they should become a permanent part of the drug surveillance system.

The remaining analytical schemes are drug-related and organised by independent agencies. The University of Southampton scheme, which is at present testing the scheme with six drugs, has the advantage that it can be applied to all N.H.S. prescriptions in England, whilst the Smith Kline & French scheme, because of its limitation to pharmacists, would only do so if the majority of pharmacists took part. The latter's scheme was limited to very large towns and, therefore, the results cannot necessarily be extrapolated to rural populations, since the standard of general practice is probably different in town and country areas.

The two schemes do not cover the same ADR, the Smith Kline & French scheme limiting enquiries to hospital diagnoses and deaths, whilst the University of Southampton scheme enquires about all events, including symptoms, that the general practitioner has recorded. The filtering out of symptoms and G.P. diagnoses will probably not reduce the efficiency of the S.K.F. scheme to any great extent but the inclusion of symptoms in the University of Southampton scheme may produce problems.

Both schemes are adequate for the search for a hypothesis but both control groups have built-in biases. The S.K.F. scheme control group is chosen

Figure 6   Types of P.M.S.

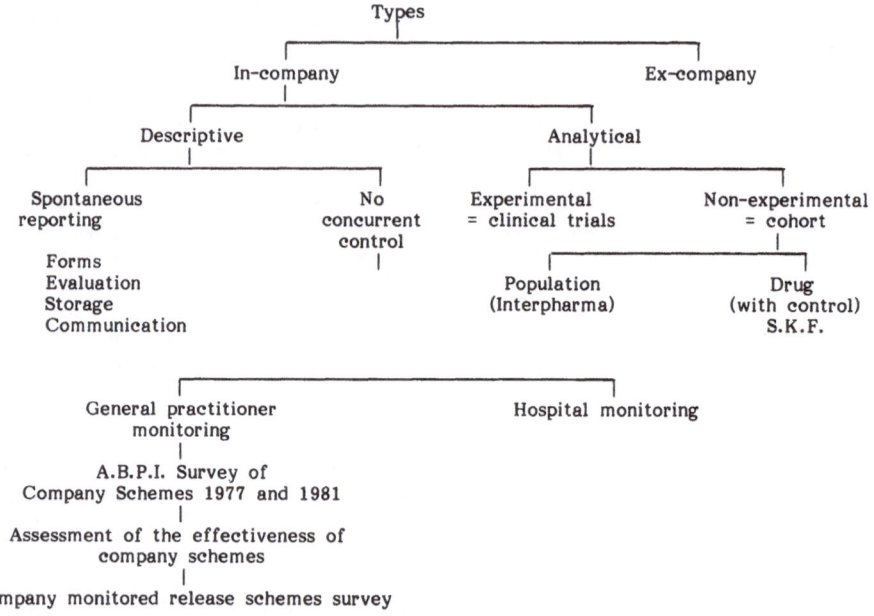

three months after the active group and is chosen - age and sex matched - from the same practice as a patient on cimetidine but does not have the same underlying disease.   If any other disease is linked with peptic ulcer disease, it may appear to be linked with the cimetidine-treated group but not the control group.   Similarly, in the University of Southampton scheme there are possible biases (see page 105).   Once a hypothesis is put forward in either scheme, a case-control study or a further study of another database, such as a record linkage scheme, will be necessary to test this hypothesis.   Methods for removing the various biases in case-control studies have been put forward[241].   The problem of examining many hypotheses has already been discussed (see page 12).

Case-control studies are the most economical means of discovering rare drug-induced diseases.

SPONTANEOUS REPORTING TO THE PHARMACEUTICAL COMPANY

Once a drug is marketed, information flows in from many sources.

Figure 7: Company sources of ADR

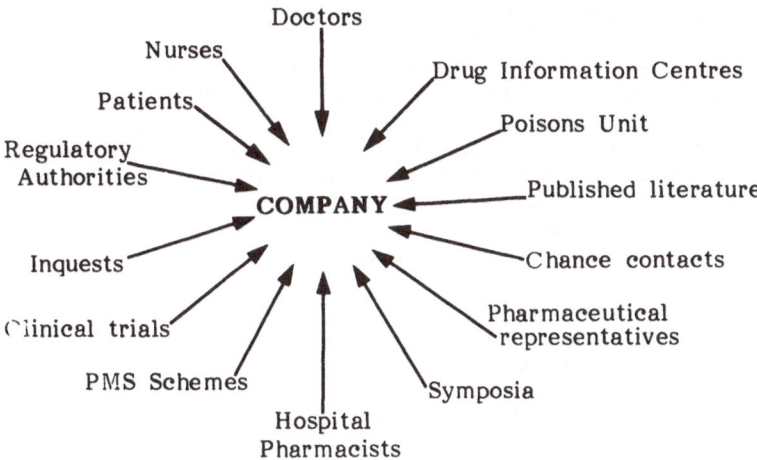

This should not be a mere passive acceptance of facts which reach the adverse reaction personnel - a positive approach is required. Everybody within the company, as well as many of the sources mentioned above, needs to be made aware that adverse event reports are welcomed and that uncertainty about their relationship is no bar to reporting. The pharmaceutical company has a source of information on possible adverse reactions that is not open to any other body and that is its sales representatives. They have regular contacts with prescribing doctors and should make the most of these opportunities by asking, "Have you heard of any possible adverse reactions to any of our products?". If there is a positive reply a company adverse reaction form can be given to the doctor with a request to give as much detail as possible.

The process of dealing with reported adverse events comes under six main headings:-

(1)   Acknowledgment and validation.

(2)   Collection of further information.

(3)   Evaluation of all data.

(4)   Action decision.

(5)   Storage of data.

(6)   Communication of results.

Acknowledgment and validation

A personal letter, thanking the source for the information is essential. In many cases it will request further information or will contain a copy of the company's adverse reaction form. Wherever possible, it should also contain further details of the company's information concerning that type of adverse reaction. Not all reports come in the form of information; one of the commonest approaches is as a request: "Can your drug cause ....?" and one must not fail to follow these up, since they nearly always have an adverse event to report.

Not all reports require validation, since this would be physically impossible. The Sandoz Company (U.S.A.) use the following criteria[245] for deciding whether a visit to the reporter is required:

(a)   Deaths attributed to any products where overdosage was believed not to be a factor.

(b)   Serious or alarming adverse experiences for any product.

(c)   Unusual experiences to any product.

These criteria apply to those events requiring validation but I believe it should also apply to accidental and suicidal overdosages.

Both tact and discretion are required in the validation of data since it can be easily mistaken for an attempt to dissociate the drug from the adverse event for commercial rather than scientific reasons. Irey has reported that of 94 adverse reaction reports sent to the Armed Forces Institute of Pathology (U.S.A.) 38% were attributed to other causes when additional data about these reports had been obtained[120]. Even when the source seems to be beyond reproach, validation is still required.

Collection of further information

The seven areas for which information is necessary for evaluation of an adverse event are, according to Dangoumau[116]:

(i)   chronology

(ii)   dechallenge

(iii)   rechallenge

(iv)   clinical symptomatology

(v)   other possible explanations

(vi)   possible predisposition

(vii)   complementary investigations

The situation after marketing is slightly different to that before marketing and the company adverse reaction form should reflect these differences.

(a)   There is no onus on the physician to fill in the company form – therefore, it must be made easy to fill in and to return, and a reasonable compromise made between brevity and adequacy.

(b)   The multitudinous sources are unlikely to be as capable or interested as those involved in clinical trials.

(c)   The form should be suitable for computerisation.

(d)   It should offer to inform regulatory authorities if the reporter has not already done so and, therefore, must cover at least the ground covered by the C.S.M.'s yellow card and the F.D.A.'s FD 1639.

Castle of I.C.I. has listed the following information as being required[246]:

1.   **Identification of Report**

Reference number, country, information source outside company, source reference (if applicable), information source inside company, date of report or adverse reaction to company, date of report to National Registration Authority (if applicable), Registration Authority concerned.

2.   **Patient particulars**

Name, town, patient's doctor, N.H.S. number (where relevant), date of birth, weight, race, occupation, sex, whether pregnant, present diagnosis, important family history, allergy.

3.   **Adverse reaction particulars**

Nature, severity, date of reaction, whether there is pathological confirmation, previous history of this reaction in this patient, other normal/abnormal clinical findings, most recent clinical state, reasons for resolution (if resolved), duration (if resolved).

4.   **Drug particulars**

Company's drug, date first prescribed, medication indication, route of administration, average daily dose, maximum daily dose (if different), duration of treatment and reaction (if applicable), time sequence between company drug and adverse reaction, number of other drugs involved, specification of other drugs, time sequence for these other drugs.

A reasonable approach to the problem of forms is to have two general forms:

Form 1 (appendix page 216): similar to the forms required by regulatory authorities, preferably folding to make a pre-paid envelope. Rather than requesting the patient's name, "patient identification" should be requested so that the doctor can choose how he identifies the patient, i.e. name or initials, Health Service number, hospital number or Hogben number (the first three letters of the surname followed by the initial of the first Christian name, a six figure date of birth and finally the initial denoting sex, i.e. STE M 240130 M). This gives the opportunity for confidentiality. On receipt of the form the patient identification should be transferred to an index and given an individual reference number. The original forms will go into the company's archives with access only by adverse reaction personnel. When a case is closed the data should be microfiched and filed separately from the original hard copy and identified only by the adverse reactions number. The index book with the only record of patient identification should be available only to named staff dealing with ADR and be under lock and key.

This form should also include asking for the opinion of the reporter in two areas:

(1)   causal relationship of the event - as far as the drug is concerned.

(2)   causal relationship of the event - as far as other possible causes are concerned.

Form 2 (appendix, page 217): A more extensive form is required to cover the additional data usually available in the more severe cases, i.e. laboratory investigations, biopsy and possible post-mortem results. This form should only be used on rare occasions at the instigation of the adverse reactions personnel. Any known details from Form 1 should be filled in prior to sending it to the doctor. This form will, on the whole, be limited to adverse events occurring in hospitals. Naturally, the simple Form 1 should not attract a fee; but, since the more extensive form requires a painstaking search of the patient's records, a fee should be paid, the level of payment being similar to that paid by an insurance company for a report.

Special forms must be designed for specific areas. These fall into two categories:

1.   Organ related, i.e. skin, psychiatry, anaesthesia. The range of a
        company's products will dictate which forms will be required.

2.   Event related. This refers to the rare adverse drug reaction which
        has not been seen before or has special characteristics. This form
        is designed with the aim of learning the maximum amount about the
        characteristics of the event, such as predisposing factors, either
        demographic or pharmacological. Since this is a specific form, it
        cannot be designed until the ADR has been recognised.

Evaluation of all data

Where an adverse event has been acknowledged previously as being an
attribution of a drug and the event is not serious and is also common with
that drug, no evaluation need be carried out. The number of events
relative to the total sales figures should give a rough incidence figure and
this must be checked at regular intervals for a change in incidence.
Adverse events associated with a drug form a continuum from the common
mild/transient side effects (Type A) to the rare, serious adverse events
Type B. The common mild/transient side effects should be discovered
before marketing by large-scale comparative studies of the new drug
compared with either placebo or standard therapy. The statistical analysis
of these studies should indicate whether or not the drug is a probable cause
of the event but will not be able to indicate whether the event in a
particular patient was due to the drug or not. On the other hand, where
there is a rare serious event, full investigation will be warranted and a
consensus of opinion - the clinician knowing most about the patient and the
event, the company expert knowing most about the drug, its pharmacology
and its previous ADR history, and the specialist in the field of the event
having the final word. The use of algorithms, decision tables and scorings
is most useful in the "mid-field" ensuring a standardised logical approach
to difficult problems.

Evaluations require investigation of the other concurrent drugs to see if
they might be responsible alone or whether a possible interaction is
involved.   The standard reference books[247], Meyler's Side Effects of
Drugs, 9th edition, plus the annual editions 4, 5, 6 and 7 are best for this
purpose.

It will be necessary to search the adverse reaction database for the
suspected drug to find whether there is a precedent for the drug/event
combination. As well as using the database, most cases will also be
referred to a company product specialist for opinion and comment. Reference may also be necessary to the company toxicologists, biochemists,
pharmacists or pharmacologists and, if the drug or a similar one is
manufactured by another company, their comments may also be sought.
Where necessary, an outside opinion from a consultant will be requested,
as mentioned earlier.

The evaluation decision may be produced in several different forms ranging, from a single word on the one event to a long report on a general adverse reaction problem.

Storage of data and Communication

These subjects are dealt with in full in Chapter 8.

COMPANY POSTMARKETING SURVEILLANCE

A breakdown of the types of postmarketing surveillance that industry has undertaken is shown in **Figure 6, page 110.**

General Practitioner Monitoring

A.B.P.I. Survey (1977) of Company Monitored Release Schemes

Sullman (1977) gave a resumé of the pharmaceutical industry's experiences with monitored release at a Medico-Pharmaceutical Forum meeting on postmarketing surveillance of adverse reactions to new medicines[248]. The resume was based on the experience of fifteen companies, eight of whom had had monitored release imposed upon them, whilst the other seven did so of their own choice. The majority were of short or medium term, i.e. three months or less. Sullman did not identify the companies and spoke only in general terms. She said that there was rarely data for more than 100 to 200 patients for two years. The drop-out rates were high but no information is given as to how these were dealt with or the reason for the high drop-out rates. As far as the success of the schemes was concerned, "new information obtained on adverse reactions had been minimal". The assessment of the cost was that it ranged from about £100,000 per 1,000 patients whether they were monitored for three months or two years. The Allen & Hanbury's research company's costs (including staff salaries, computerisation etc) was in agreement with her general estimate. Of the monitored release type schemes that have been mentioned in the literature 53 have given the number of patients involved and, based on Sullman's figures, these schemes have cost at least 33 million pounds.

A.B.P.I. Survey (1981) of Company Monitored Release Schemes[248]

During the summer of 1981 the A.B.P.I. sent out questionnaires to 85 companies on postmarketing studies operated since 1st January 1977. Twenty-eight companies (68%) replied; 38 of these had not done any such studies and 17 had done some sort of scheme. Of the 18 schemes operated (one company had conducted two schemes) 11 were initiated voluntarily by the company, 5 were started as a result of a request from the Licensing Authority and only 2 schemes were commenced as a requirement of the

U.K. licence. Each of the 18 schemes was conducted by the company. The information was given by the A.B.P.I. without disclosing the names of the companies. The A.B.P.I. report is now an historic document and does not necessarily represent current procedures. (see appendix pages 210-211).

Assessment of the effectiveness of company-initiated PMS

An effective PMS should be able to:

(1)   Confirm and quantify all previously known ADR.

(2)   If any previously unknown ADR are discovered as a result of PMS, then these should be confirmed subsequently.

(3)   If no new ADR is discovered during the PMS, then none should be discovered by other means either during or after the PMS within the limits set by the numbers involved in the PMS.

Method

Each of these aims will be examined in turn.

Confirm and quantify all previously known ADR

The previously known ADR are divided into the two types (page 15) specific and non-specific. Specific ADR are much rarer than non-specific ADR but, if they do occur, then provided that the PMS is efficient these will be recognised and their discovery will be a function of the number of patients involved, the time to onset of the ADR and the duration of the PMS. However, few specific ADR are immediately recognisable as being such but will more often masquerade as naturally occurring disease until intensive investigation reveals their true nature. The time from the first symptoms of the latter type until the final recognition of its relationship to the drug will vary from weeks to many months and may, therefore, only be recognised after the PMS is over unless all patients under investigation at the end of the survey period are followed up - an immense task, not mentioned as having been undertaken in any of the schemes.

There is no reason to believe that any of the PMS schemes would not have detected and quantified any previously known ADR of the specific type as long as the time to recognition fell within the duration of the scheme. This then is a strong point of company initiated schemes and can be exemplified by the Pfizer Hypovase Syncope Scheme[249]. Non-specific ADR (having a naturally occurring incidence) will not be accurately quantified without a randomised control group and, since no scheme incorporated the latter, none can accurately quantify any known ADR.

A task force set up by the F.D.A. has reviewed a selection of Phase 4[238] studies and their contribution to postmarketing surveillance.   The PMS schemes selected were the U.S.A. cimetidine, cyclobenzapine and prazosin studies.   The review has been published in a shortened form[250] and also as a longer, more critical document[251].   The latter gave the following conclusions.

(1)   Phase 4 studies as carried out in the past are not likely to lead to the discovery of new adverse reactions.

(2)   Confirmatory studies of incidence rates for already known and commonly occuring ADR in Phase 4 studies are likely to demonstrate qualitative and quantitative differences from those seen in the clinical trials.   (The incidence of ADR in the PMS was far lower than those recorded for placebo patients in clinical trials.)

(3)   Alternative strategies for carrying out Phase 4 studies should be considered if Phase 4 studies remain an important PMS objective.

(4)   A better defined and more formal administrative framework for sponsor/F.D.A. interaction in Phase 4 studies should be worked out before many more new, important and potentially costly Phase 4 studies are initiated.

This document should be read in conjunction with an I.M.S. document "An experiment in early postmarketing surveillance of drugs" in order to have a good understanding of the American experience.

If any previously unknown ADR are discovered as a result of PMS then these should be confirmed subsequently

Two cases of haematemesis occurring in patients with a history of gastric ulcer in a small PMS scheme resulted in a change in the data sheet and these changes persist in the 1984 data sheet[252].   Doctors will, therefore, have been discouraged from prescribing in similar cases.   Those who prescribed this drug despite this reservation and produced a further haematemesis are unlikely to report, either because it is in the data sheet already or because of it being a confession of negligence.   Either way no further reports are likely, so it will never be known whether these were two isolated cases occurring by chance or whether it is a true ADR.   This is the penalty of early publication of a possible ADR.

If no ADR are discovered during the PMS schemes, then none should be discovered by other means either during or after the PMS scheme (within the limits imposed by the number of patients in each scheme)

It is necessary to examine a large number of these schemes and then search the literature for subsequent newly discovered ADR.   The F.D.A. survey   mentioned above examined three studies and acknowledged that the ADR discovered outside the PMS may have been of such rarity that they were unlikely to be discovered in the schemes due to lack of numbers. We need, therefore, to survey a much larger selection of PMS studies if we are to estimate the capability of company PMS schemes to discover new ADR.

Company monitored release schemes

This is defined here as any postmarketing scheme organised by a pharmaceutical company in which one of the main aims is to establish the safety or tolerance of the drug and in which there is no randomised concurrent control group, the number of patients involved to exceed one hundred.

Since 1970 many companies have initiated monitored release schemes. Sixty of these schemes have been reviewed[253] and data on 25 have been published. Only three of the schemes had a control group. There is no mention in any of these publications of a newly discovered ADR (with one exception, see page 118). The total number of patients involved in 57 of these schemes was 340,346 and, based on Sullman's minimum estimate of costs, the total cost would be approximately £34 million. The earlier schemes have tended to report side effects whilst the later schemes report adverse events. Eight of these schemes were monitoring for specific ADR.

The 60 schemes represent eleven countries, as follows: U.K. 31, U.S.A. 10, Germany 3, Italy 4, France 2, Canada 2, Norway, Sweden, Finland, Japan and South Africa one each and three multi-national schemes. The duration of these schemes is shown in the table below. In 41 of these schemes there was either a statement to the effect that no new ADR had been discovered or the paper gave a detailed account of the scheme without any mention of the discovery of any new ADR. Subsequent to the PMS or parallel to it there were 106 spontaneously reported cases of adverse events associated with the 25 drugs involved. Rossi et al[250] have examined the American PMS schemes of three drugs, cimetidine, prazosin and cyclo-benzapine (these were also examined in the author's survey). Four new ADR were published subsequent to the prazosin scheme, 17 ADR or interactions for cimetidine and none for cyclobenzapine.

Duration	1/52	1/12	2/12	3/12	1 yr.	2 yrs.	3 yrs.	Not Stated
Number	2	11	6	11	9	6	4	10

Many factors may be responsible for the failure to detect ADR during these PMS schemes:

(a) **Possible ADR were discovered but not published**

Since causal relationships cannot be demonstrated in uncontrolled studies unless there is individual positive rechallenge (a great rarity in general practice) only hypotheses could have been generated. If then a reasonable decision was made by the company not to publish hypotheses and no further evidence was generated to prove or disprove the hypothesis, then this would account for the failure to detect ADR.

(b) **Lack of numbers**

Lack of numbers in the PMS relative to the incidence of the subsequently discovered ADR. This may be a factor in many of these schemes but it is very unlikely that all 106 hypotheses had incidences such that none of them would have been found in the 41 schemes.

(c) **Brevity**

This may well be a factor in many of the schemes since the majority lasted for three months or less and many ADR only become manifest after more than three months' treatment.

(d) **Causal relationship demanded before reporting**

If the protocol for a PMS scheme requires reporting of side effects or adverse drug reactions or any similar term, it will suggest that only those adverse events which the clinician believes to be drug-related will be reported. Those protocols requesting adverse event reporting should have avoided this factor.

(e) **Delay in recognition of ADR**

PMS usually only involves G.P.s. Lack of experience and facilities are not in favour of the recognition of ADR by G.P.s compared with specialist hospital staff. Since most serious diseases are passed to the hospital service for diagnosis and initial treatment, the serious ADR will most likely be recognised by the hospital service. The delay between the presentation to the G.P. of the ADR, the decision to refer the patient for a further opinion, delay in N.H.S. appointments and possible hospital admission or investigation and the subsequent delay in informing the G.P. of the results are quite likely to take the patient beyond the duration of the PMS

(f) **Relative efficiency of pre-marketing clinical trials (PMCT) compared with PMS**

PMCT are expected to recognise ADR with an incidence of up to 1 in 100. PMS (6,000 to 10,000 patients) is expected to identify ADR with an incidence of up to 1 in 1,000. If PMS schemes are ten times less efficient in picking up rare side effects than PMCT, the PMS will not be able to improve on the 1:100 detection by PMCT since they will cover the same incidence of ADR. The factor of time could **alone explain the lack of success of PMS (see appendix page 233, comparison of PMCT and PMS studies).**

Since PMCT and PMS cover all types of drugs, diseases and patients, the table contains only generalisations which are difficult to substantiate and many of them are a matter of opinion. Company initiated PMS schemes have no advantage when compared with PMCT plus spontaneous reporting with the exception that they can quantify specific ADR discovered during PMCT.

I believe that pharmaceutical companies should not undertake uncontrolled cohort studies for the purpose of discovering previously unknown adverse reactions, for the following reasons:

1. There is no evidence that company PMS schemes are capable of detecting new ADR.

2. No company can employ sufficient numbers of trained staff to deal with the peak of activitiy without have superfluous trained staff in the interim period.

3. No one company will have sufficient continuing experience to advance methodology.

4. No company will be prepared or be able to monitor a similar sized control group on another company's product.

5. Many company PMS schemes have been disguised "seeding trials" and discredit the industry.

6. The reputation of the pharmaceutical industry in the field of adverse drug reactions is so tarnished that its statements carry little weight.

This is not to say that some of the more recent PMS schemes organised by companies and which monitored adverse events would not have detected ADR occurring within the range governed by the numbers involved.

I believe that pharmaceutical companies are best suited to arranging longterm multicentre hospital based, randomly allocated controlled studies between their new drug and standard therapy with active monitoring for adverse events. Uncontrolled cohort studies should be restricted to those with the specific aim of finding out more about previously discovered ADR. Studies for the detection of new ADR in the postmarketing period without randomly allocated controls would be best organised by outside agencies such as Dr. Inman's Prescription Event Monitoring, Professor Langman's study group or the R.C.G.P. postmarketing surveillance group.

Hospital monitoring

Since there are many drugs which are almost exclusively used in hospital there will be occasions when a hospital monitoring PMS is essential. These PMS schemes will resemble the pre-marketing uncontrolled studies in hospital and will present similar problems in their evaluation. There are also many drugs which are prescribed both in general practice and in hospital in-patient practice and in these cases two separate PMS schemes (hospital and general practice) would complement each other.

In-company analytical studies

Experimental (clinical trials)

These can be divided into two groups depending upon the subject and the clinical trialists:

(1)   In patients conducted by physicians outside the company

(2)   In volunteers conducted by physicians within the company

In patients conducted by physicians outside the company

There should be little difference between the clinical trials before and after marketing except that after marketing there will be more general practitioner trials. The newly agreed rules governing these trials should improve both the scientific and ethical quality of these studies. In the U.K. postmarketing general practice studies should conform to the code of practice drawn up by the British Medical Association (B.M.A.), the Royal College of General Practice and the ABPI. Clause 5.13 deals with adverse reactions:[254]

> "The method of follow-up assessment and investigation of suspected adverse reactions must be described. Investigators must be reminded of the obligation to use their supplies of yellow cards to notify the Committe on Safety of Medicines (DHSS, Medicines Division, Market Towers, 1 Nine Elms Lane, London SW8 5NQ) of serious or unusual adverse reactions to any medicinal product and of all adverse reactions to a new medicinal product and to inform the company medical adviser. The company medical adviser has an obligation to inform the Committee on Safety of Medicines of adverse drug reactions and must also, when appropriate, inform other investigators of any serious or unusual adverse reaction."

In volunteers conducted by physicians within the company

Only common side effects are likely to be seen during the phase 1 and 2 studies in volunteers due to the small number involved.

Non-experimental analytical studies

These may be of two types:

(1)   Case-control studies/case studies

(2)   Cohort studies

The former are not usually arranged by the industry since the unusual diagnoses or adverse events will occur only in patients. The only example where this type of study has been arranged has been by Castle of I.C.I. who arranged a study of Peyronie's disease because there was considerable doubt as to whether this could be caused by beta-blocking drugs[243].

Cohort studies can be arranged either by population group or drug oriented studies.   There is only one cohort study based on a hospital population which is affiliated to the pharmaceutical industry and that is the Interpharma System in Berne, Switzerland.   This is a co-operative venture between Professor Hoigne of Zieglerspital and the three pharmaceutical companies in Basle: F Hoffman-La Roche, Ciba-Geigy and Sandoz Ltd. Bruppacher of F Hoffman-La Roche has described his company's involvement but no details of any new adverse reaction discovered by this means have been published, so the assessment of this scheme is not possible[255].

For reasons mentioned earlier it is unlikely that a pharmaceutical company will undertake a cohort study with a control group other than placebo. Smith Kline & French have collaborated with Lawson in the monitoring of cimetidine with such a study, as has already been mentioned[233].

An alternative design which should be considered more frequently is a randomised study comparing the new drug with the drug which the consultant would normally use, i.e. his own standard therapy. This control group would be heterogeneous in that there would be many different choices for the control drug, but it can be argued that the comparison would be valid and ethical and the number of patients available for the study would be greatly increased. This design would overcome one of the main problems of hospital monitoring, i.e. the small number of patients available.

Update

In human Toxicology (1984) 3,261-269. "Inherent Limitations of the Yellow Card System for the Detection of Unsuspected Adverse Drug Reactions". I. Crombie points out that hospital doctors are better placed for detecting new ADR than general practitioners and suggests that a modified yellow card system designed to encourage reporting by hospital clinicians could be of greater value than the present system. This paper, contains interesting data to support this hypothesis.

CONCLUSIONS

Postmarketing surveillance must be welded to the pre-marketing surveillance for ADR.   Controlled clinical trials of the same calibre as those organised by the original research team will continue.   Although all clinical trials have some marketing advantage, all of them should be able to stand on their own scientific feet.   Uncontrolled large-scale G.P. studies with an aim of discovering any previously unknown ADR should be avoided.   The spontaneous reporting part of PMS needs to be very flexible if the maximum amount of information is to be gained from it.   Any step that makes it easier for the observer of a possible ADR to report it to the company should be taken, including the use of a standard question by the pharmaceutical representative.   PMS is a continuing process which never ceases and is largely in the hands of the pharmaceutical company.   The most useful tool in the hands of the company is the large randomised controlled clinical trial comparing the new drug with standard therapy. Studies without randomised controls should be carried out by independent authorities with the maximum of co-operation from the company

6
Drug Rechallenge

It is generally agreed that the result of a drug rechallenge is the most important single factor in ascribing causality[256,257]. The manner in which it is performed is crucial and considerable thought needs to be given to it.

Definition

The giving of a further dose(s) of a drug to a person who had previously taken a dose(s) of the same drug and in whom an adverse event, which might be due to that drug, had subsequently occurred.

Accidental drug rechallenge

Adverse events are always occurring during drug treatment and the process of relating the event to the drug has been discussed. There are many occasions, however, when the possibility of a relationship is neither considered by the patient nor by the doctor and a further dose of the drug is taken in the course of the previously prescribed treatment. The recurrence of the event with the subsequent doses may then be recognised retrospectively as being related to the drug or the possibility considered If the relationship is doubtful, a further deliberate rechallenge may be considered.

Deliberate drug rechallenge

If an adverse event has occurred during or after drug treatment and the possibility that the event is related to the drug has been considered by the prescribing doctor, then he will consider whether or not a further dose(s) should be given. There are many factors that he will need to consider before making that decision.

Ethics

The first question to be answered is "How will the patient benefit from the rechallenge?" It may be that it is the patient alone who will benefit or it may be that all future patients for whom this drug is considered would profit from knowing whether or not the drug is the cause of the event.   In the latter case future patients may profit either directly, i.e. their own treatment will be affected by the knowledge that the event and the drug are or are not related, or they may benefit indirectly in that the rechallenge may add to our knowledge of the mechanism of the reaction and this may aid future research into other drugs.   There must be a clear distinction between the benefit/cost ratio decision for the patient suffering the adverse event and any possible benefit to future patients. This will be considered under two separate headings.

Possible benefit to the original patient

This requires the doctor to assess the possible benefits of rechallenge against its possible risks.   If the possible benefits outweigh the possible risks, then there are no ethical problems.

Possible benefits to future patients

There may be occasions when the possible benefits to future patients will be sufficient to warrant asking the patient to run the risks and discomforts of rechallenge.   In these circumstances the binding oath of the Declaration of Geneva of the World Medical Association "the health of my patient will be my first consideration" must be considered in the context of the Declaration of Helsinki.

The first consideration must be whether the study is ethical. Few doctors have published their views and then only on rechallenge without qualification as to whether it was for the patient's benefit.   Suitable criteria might be:

1.   that the study is done in such a manner that the results are valid,

2.   that the relationship of the drug to the event has not already been convincingly established,

3.   that there is no reason to believe that any permanent sequelae are possible,

4.   that there is a reasonable supposition that the event will not be more unpleasant or dangerous than the original event.

It is my opinion that under these circumstances it would be ethical to ask the patient whether they would be prepared to undergo a rechallenge, having given the patient all the necessary information.

Having considered the already mentioned criteria and being of the opinion that it would be ethical to ask the patient for their informed consent, then this should be sought in writing. Is there any reason to seek approval of an ethical committee? If the doctor was certain that there would be no sequelae, that the adverse event after rechallenge would not be worse than the original event, that the trial would be valid and that the question had not already been answered, then, if the doctor was able to ask for the patient's consent in such a way that the patient could express his true wishes in the matter, I believe that no third party need be involved. However, rarely - if ever - will these latter criteria be met. If an ethical committee had to give its sanction on a rechallenge, as is the case in the U.S.A., the delay involved would probably deter many physicians from considering rechallenge. Many possible adverse reactions are reported at busy outpatient departments where there are already strong deterrents to considering anything that would delay the clinic and, if a rechallenge for an inpatient was likely to delay his discharge, this would again be a strong deterrent to rechallenge. A suitable compromise might be the immediate referral of the patient to the clinical pharmacologist or to the specialist in the field of the adverse event who would not only add his specialist opinion and arrange the rechallenge but also have the power of an ethical veto.

Incidence of rechallenge

Rechallenge is only performed occasionally. Ciba-Geigy[258] have stated that in less than 5% of the adverse events reported to them was rechallenge undertaken, whilst the Pharmacovigilance centre in Bordeaux[138] reports that their rechallenge rate was 4.4%.

Partial rechallenge

There are occasions when complete stopping of a drug is not justified and reduction in dosage suffices either to stop the adverse reaction or to make a significant reduction in its effect. Subsequent re-introduction of the original dosage may then rank as a rechallenge.

Factors to be considered before rechallenge[259]

1. **The patient**

    (a) The possible effect of the rechallenge on the patient's physical and mental state.

    (b) The possible effect of the patient's physical and mental state on the rechallenge.

    If the rechallenge if left too long after the adverse event, the physical or mental state of the patient may have changed and an interaction between the disease and drug missed.

2. **The underlying disease(s)**

    The disease requiring treatment may vary from a transient symptom, scarcely justifying the original drug treatment, to a life-threatening disease. The former would probably not justify rechallenge in the patient's interest and the latter may warrant rechallenge, even if the rechallenge itself could be life-threatening.

3.   **Alternative treatments**

Where there are alternative and equally efficacious treatments for the underlying disease which carry less risk than the rechallenge with the original drug, then rechallenge would not be justified for that patient's benefit.   However, it may be that the alternative treatments work through the same basic mechanism as the original drug so that their use may be the equivalent to a rechallenge but perhaps with a diminished chance of the adverse event occurring. Where there is no worthwhile alternative treatment to the original drug, then the justification for rechallenge in the patient's interest will depend on the underlying disease and the risk of rechallenge.

4.   **The original adverse event**

(a)   Cause

The relationship between the original event and the drug may vary from almost certain cause to most unlikely cause. Obviously, the less likely the drug is as the cause of the event, the less risk there is in the rechallenge and vice versa.

(b)   Severity

The assessment of the severity of the original symptoms and risk to the patient of the original event can only give a rough guide to the possible severity of the rechallenge and this will be dealt with further, when the mechanisms of the reaction are discussed.

(c)   Time to onset

When the time to onset is only a few seconds (following an intravenous injection), then the relationship to the drug is usually obvious and definite, but when the time to onset is long, the relationship is less obvious and will relate to the mechanism of the reaction, e.g. if the drug took two years to produce the original reaction, would it be necessary to continue the rechallenge for two years before saying that it was negative?

(d)   Dechallenge

Once the drug is stopped, the original reaction must disappear completely (i.e. 100% reversibility) before any rechallenge but the longer the manifestation takes to disappear on the whole, the less justifiable is rechallenge. If the time to onset and the time to its disappearance are both long, then this will weigh against rechallenge. There is an exception to the rule in that on occasions the drug dose is reduced rather than stopped with some subsidence of the adverse event and then a return to the previous dose may produce recurrence of the adverse event.

(e)   The organ system affected

Many organ systems have a limited number of responses to
drug insults and so, as the pattern of an adverse event
develops, previous examples give us some idea of the prognosis. However, we must be alert for possible new adverse
reactions. A specialist in the affected organ may need to be
consulted before a rechallenge decision is taken.

(f)   Adverse reaction mechanisms

The probable mechanism of the adverse event, if known, may
be a guide to the reproducability of the event on rechallenge.
Some reactions may increase in severity on rechallenge
(hypersensitisation) and others may decrease (desensitisation).
Any adverse event mediated by a hypersensitivity mechanism
is likely to be unpredictable on rechallenge, necessitating
either rechallenge with very small doses and/or another route
of administration. Inherent unpredictability is a contra-
indication to rechallenge when the rechallenge is not in the
patient's own interest.

(g)   The history of the drug

Where rechallenge will not benefit the patient concerned, the
degree to which rechallenge might benefit future patients will
depend on what is known concerning that drug and the event.
Previous positive rechallenge in other patients may make
further rechallenge unnecessary and unethical. When a
rechallenge is contemplated and no benefit foreseen for the
patient, the pharmaceutical company responsible for the
original research on the drug should be asked whether any
information is known about the relationship between the drug
and the event before rechallenge is undertaken.

(h)   Treatment of the adverse event

In many cases the original adverse event will require treatment and this will distort the significance of dechallenge. Only
after the treatment and the original drug have been stopped
and a period allowed for possible re-emergence of the adverse
event can rechallenge be considered. If the treatment of the
adverse event produces immediate remission of the event, the
risk for the patient will be diminished in any rechallenge.

Methods of rechallenge

1.   Blinding

In most cases where rechallenge is for the patient's benefit the
adverse event will have either objective signs/abnormal laboratory
investigations in addition to symptoms and in these cases blinding is
not so essential. However, where the adverse event consists of

subjective symptoms only and rechallenge is for the benefit of future patients, then the rechallenge should be performed using an identical placebo. If the placebo and active drug rechallenge are treated as two separate events, the patient has a 50% chance of being right by guess-work. It is, therefore, preferable, when the time to onset and offset is short, to insert the active drug period into a longer placebo period.

2.   **Dosage**

In most cases the rechallenge dosage should be similar to the original drug dosage and continue for longer than the previous time to onset to validate a negative rechallenge. Where the initial reaction was severe and a positive rechallenge is likely, then it is sensible to use a reduced dosage and be prepared to increase the dose if there is no response. Where the event is thought to be a Type A (augmented response), then the possibility of taking blood samples for drug levels should be considered. These may vary from an isolated peak blood level value to a modified dose response curve. The same dosage route should be used.

3.   **Location**

The location of the rechallenge will depend on where the original adverse event took place and the expected severity of any rechallenge event. The latter may need to be treated urgently, so rechallenge should not be performed unless adequate staff, drugs and equipment are available.

4.   **Interactions**

Since an adverse event may be the result of an interaction between the drug and disease, food, physiological state or another drug, it will be important to have only one variable under test at a time. The classical interaction study design for two drugs is a latin square design with the periods randomly allocated with, if necessary, wash-out periods. However, the underlying disease may make a double placebo period unethical.

Figure 8 INTERACTION STUDY

Placebo A	Placebo A
Active B	Placebo B

Active A	Active A
Placebo B	Active B

5.   **Multiple rechallenge**

Where it is thought that there is a possibility that a drug-related event has occurred but there is more than one candidate drug, rechallenge with each drug may be required.

6.   **Re-rechallenge**

If the first rechallenge is accidental or if a positive rechallenge is considered very unlikely and the first rechallenge is performed without the proper means of identifying the rechallenge event, a further rechallenge may be required[260]. Due consideration should again be given to the possibility of increased sensitisation or decreased sensitisation. There still remains a possibility that, although the first rechallenge is reversible, a second rechallenge may be less so[261].

Interpretation

Although a positive rechallenge is probably the strongest proof of a causal relationship, there are occasions when the results of a rechallenge can be misleading, and this is where there are possible interactions with either (a) other drugs or treatment, (b) variability of the underlying disease, (c) the patient's personality, (d) the weather, diet, etc., or where there is a possibility of desensitization taking place between the original event and the rechallenge[262].

Interaction with underlying disease can occur when the disease is very variable, e.g. cardio-selective beta-blockers may increase the severity of an asthma attack. Subsequent rechallenge when the patient is without clinical asthma and with only minimal sympathetic drive may not produce an attack, but a subsequent asthma attack occurring whilst still on the drug may be life-threatening.

Similarly, a drug may interact with the patient's personality and in the case of a placebo reactor it must be remembered that a placebo can produce objective changes, as well as subjective symptoms, hence the frequent need for a placebo control. Variable climatic conditions and Raynaud's syndrome may interact with beta-blockers to produce misleading results on rechallenge and, similarly, M.A.O.I.s used in depression can interact with some items in the diet. The possibility of unintended desensitization giving rise to a false negative dechallenge is probably very rare and difficult to substantiate.

Another false positive can be as the result of a protopathic bias; that is, the drug is given for the early symptoms of a disease which follows its course and the deterioration is considered the adverse event. Recurrence of the disease treated in the same way might be considered as a positive rechallenge.

Involvement of the pharmaceutical physician

The pharmaceutical physician may be involved with rechallenge in the following ways:

(1)   In volunteers in phase 1 studies conducted in the firm's clinical pharmacology department.

(2)   The writing of a protocol for the rechallenge of patients who develop adverse events during clinical trials.

(3)   Advising clinicians of previous experiences of rechallenge with their drugs or assessing other evidence relevant to a rechallenge.

(4)   Arranging for measurement of drug levels.

(5)   Providing placebo tablets for rechallenge.

(6)   Arranging for a panel of consultants to be available for consultation by physicians wishing to rechallenge patients. Regretfully, there is little literature published on risks involved in rechallenge relevant to the various organ systems, although there are numerous references to anecdotal cases.

Conclusion

Rechallenge should be used more frequently in premarketing clinical trials. Trialists should be encouraged to consider rechallenge in those cases where the event is a non-serious symptom without risk of sequelae. Reference should be made to this in the trial protocol which should also give details of the procedures to be followed.

7
The Regulations Concerning Adverse Reactions

INTRODUCTION

It is essential that the central organisation of a pharmaceutical company collects suspected adverse reactions associated with its products from all over the world. The laws in each country will differ and even minor differences in drug regulations will alter the quality and quantity of the adverse reactions reported to the central organisation. It is unrealistic to believe that the provision of a standard adverse reaction form and instruction to each overseas company will result in a homogeneous database. However, standardisation must be attempted. This chapter highlights the main regulations in the six most important world markets - United States of America, Japan, France, Germany, Italy and the United Kingdom. However, it is no substitute for the study of the original regulations, when appropriate. Since the United States is the most profitable market in the world, its requirements in the field of drug safety tend to dominate the thoughts of pharmaceutical companies.

The recent problems with benoxaprofen, zomepirac and Osmosin have highlighted various deficiencies in the laws concerning adverse drug reaction reporting. The suggested new changes in U.S.A. law are outlined here. The U.K. will have a revised MAL 2 and MAL 4 during 1984. The French Ministry of Health is considering the introduction of obligatory reporting of adverse reactions.

UNITED KINGDOM

Legal requirements concerning ADR

At present in the U.K. the Medicines Act, 1968, governs the reporting of ADR by the pharmaceutical industry. The Secretaries of State respectively concerned with health in England, Wales and Scotland have the power under section 47(1) of the Medicines Act, 1968 (a), to make regulations, one of which is the Medicines (Standard Provisions for Licences and Certificates) Regulations 1971.

133

Regulations concerning pre-marketing trials

The above regulation in Schedule 1 Part II, Regulation 3(2), paragraph 2 deals with the reporting of adverse reactions while the clinical trial certificate is in force.

"2.   The certificate holder shall forthwith inform the licensing authority of any information received by him that casts doubt on the continued validity of the data which was submitted with, or in connection with, the application for the clinical trial certificate for the purpose of being taken into account in assessing the safety, quality or efficacy of any medicinal products to which the certificate relates for the purpose for which the certificate holder proposed that it may be used."

The regulations for the subsequent reporting of adverse drug reactions which occur in those trials carried out under a clinical trials certificate are contained in "Notes on application for Product Licences, MAL 2, D.H.S.S., May 1977, Part IV, Studies in Humans":

1.   Human Pharmacological Studies

   If studies have been undertaken in volunteers they must be reported if they have any relevance to the drug's safety.

2.   Where a product is to be administered on a long-term basis, evidence of the long-term efficacy in a substantial number of patients is needed.

   2.1   Summary of all clinical trials

      2.1.7   Adverse reactions - all to be reported whether major or minor.

      2.2.3   Details and reasons for patients withdrawn before the end of the treatment period must be stated.

      2.3.8   Reports of suspected drug dependence (including habituation, addiction or difficulty in weaning patients off the drug) or interactions must be submitted in detail.

3.   Adverse reactions

   Any information available on adverse reactions reporting during clinical use of the drug in any country. A commentary on these reports may be helpful: it should assess the extent of adverse reactions reporting in the countries concerned. Individual case reports are not required unless the reactions were severe or of an unusual nature.

When an exemption from a clinical trials certificate has been applied for and no objections raised according to The Medicines (Exemption from

Licences) (Clinical Trials) Order 1981 (S1 1981 No. 164) the phraseology is somewhat different.

Stage 1:   "This would involve early searching, heavily monitored clinical pharmacological studies in limited numbers of patients.

Stage 2:   ...... open clinical studies ...... to provide information on short-term safety and acceptability and tolerance".

The Statutory Instrument 1981 No. 164 details the clinical trial exemption scheme and here the exemption holder has to make certain undertakings regarding adverse reactions and drug safety, i.e. to notify the licensing authority of effects associated with the administration of the medicinal product:

6.1.1   any adverse reaction arising during the trial.

6.1.2   any other matters coming to their attention that might reasonably cause the Licensing Authority to think that the medicinal product could no longer be regarded as a product which could safely be administered for the purpose of the clinical trial ...."

and in MAL 62, page 7, 4.1.2, the paragraph above is shortened to "any other matter that might reasonably cause the licensing authority to doubt the safety or quality of the product in question".

Regulations concerning marketed drugs

The relevant sections are Schedule 1, part 1, paragraphs 3 and 4 of the Medicines (Standard Provisions for Licences and Certificates) Regulations 1971:

3.   The licence holder shall forthwith inform the licensing authority of any information received by him that casts doubt on the continued validity of the data which was submitted with, or in connection with, the application for the product licence for the purpose of being taken into account in assessing the safety, quality or efficacy of any medicinal product to which the licence relates.

4.   The licence holder shall maintain a record of reports, of which he is aware, of adverse effects in one or more human beings associated in those reports with the use of any medicinal product to which the licence relates, which shall be open to inspection by a person authorised by the licensing authority, who may take copies thereof, and if the licensing authority so directs, the licence holder shall furnish the licensing authority with a copy of any such reports of which he has a record or of which he is or subsequently becomes aware.

The licence holder for each drug is also given directions for the reporting of adverse reactions for each drug.   The standard direction sheet is as follows:

MEDICINES ACT 1968

DIRECTION AS TO REPORTING OF SUSPECTED ADVERSE REACTIONS

Holder of the Licence ....

1.   In pursuance of para 4 Part I of Schedule 1 to the Medicines Act
       (Standard Provisions for Licences and Certificates) Regulations 1971
       (SI 1971 No. 972) as applied to any product licence held by the holder
       of the licence named above, the licensing authority directs the holder
       of the licence to furnish to the authority for the information of the
       Committee on Safety of Medicines, except where the holder of the
       licence has already furnished the Committee with the information
       and received an acknowledgment, copies of all reports, as defined in
       2 below and originating in the United Kingdom, of which he is aware
       of adverse effects on human beings suspected of association with the
       use of any medicinal product to which any such licence relates. The
       holder of the licence is required to furnish such reports as soon as
       possible after receipt or, where appropriate, immediately after
       substantiation by the patient's doctor. Licence holders should ensure
       that in all cases such reports are furnished not later than one month
       after receipt.

2.   This direction applies to any report made by or confirmed by a
       medical or dental practitioner, a pharmacist, a coroner or a
       procurator fiscal and which relates to an adverse effect which has
       occurred at doses in normal use and falls within one or more of the
       following categories:

       a.   a reaction with a fatal outcome,

       b.   a reaction of sufficient severity to interfere with normal
              activities,

       c.   any unusual reaction, not referred to in standard publication or
              in literature issued by the manufacturer or licence holder,

       d.   any reaction which may be an example of possible drug-
              interaction.

3.   The holder of the licence is also required similarly to furnish without
       delay information from abroad of which he becomes aware about
       suspected adverse reactions to medicinal products of the kind to
       which the licence relates, that is containing the same active
       ingredients, which suggests that an associated serious hazard may
       exist.   Separate reports of every relevant individual suspected
       adverse effect occurring abroad coming to the notice of the holder
       of the licence are, however, not required.

4.   This direction is without prejudice to any specific direction made in
       connection with a particular product and remains in force until

withdrawn or amended by a fresh notification in writing by the licensing authority.

Accompanying the standard direction there is a list of requirements as to reporting of suspected adverse reactions. The most important paragraphs are 2 and 7:

2.   In the case of new products a direction will be made requiring all suspected reactions originating in the United Kingdom to be reported until further notice. For all other products the direction will relate only to serious or unexpected reactions. (The direction will also require relevant information from abroad to be reported, but not in the form of copies of individual reports, and only if that information suggests a potentially important hazard may exist).

7.   The following are examples of reactions which should always be regarded as serious and should therefore be reported in all cases:

Anaphylaxis	Severe CNS effects
Blood dyscrasias	Severe skin reactions after injection or topical application
Congenital abnormalities	Reactions in pregnant women
Endocrine disturbances	Unexplained lack of effect or
Fertility effects	paradoxical effects:
Haemorrhage from any site	e.g. possibility of reduction in
Jaundice, however mild	efficacy due to drug-interaction,
Ophthalmic signs or symptoms	or hypertension with a hypotensive agent

Any symptoms of a serious or life-threatening disease which was not present before the patient was treated with the drug and any significant worsening of a concurrent condition not regarded as an indication for treatment with the drug in question.

Paragraph 2, page 136, referring to the directions for new products is given in more details in a special direction sheet which is identical but with the following phrases omitted:

Paragraph 2:   "and which relates .... example of possible drug interaction".

Paragraph 4:   "is without prejudice .... possible product and"

In October 1983 the Committee on Safety of Medicines (C.S.M.) [Market Towers, 1 Nine Elms Lane, London SW8 5NQ] published in their leaflet "Current Problems, No. 12" a more detailed account of the suspected adverse reactions which should be reported to the C.S.M. by the doctor looking after the patient:

"Suspected adverse reactions to any therapeutic agent should be reported. These agents include drugs, vaccines, blood products, X-ray contrast media, dental or surgical materials, IUCDs, absorbable sutures and contact lens fluids.

Newer drugs: (marked ▼ in the Data Sheet Compendium, BNF and MIMS). Doctors are asked to report any adverse or unexpected event, however minor, which could conceivably be attributed to the drug. Reports should be made despite uncertainty in the doctor's mind about a causal relationship, irrespective of whether the reaction is well recognised, and even if other drugs have been given concurrently.

Established drugs: Doctors are asked to report any suspected adverse drug reaction which was potentially dangerous, incapacitating or lethal. These should be reported even though the toxic effect is well recognised. Examples include anaphylaxis, blood dyscrasias, endocrine disturbances, effects on fertility, haemorrhage from any site, renal impairment, jaundice, ophthalmic disorders, severe CNS effects, severe skin reactions, reactions in pregnant women, and any drug interactions. For established drugs, doctors are asked not to report well-known, relatively minor side effects, such as dry mouth with tricyclic antidepressants, constipation with opiates, or nausea with digoxin. The reason for seeking reports of well-known but serious adverse reactions to established drugs is to enable comparisons to be made of relative risk/benefit between different drugs of similar classes.

Special problems

1.   Delayed drug effects. Doctors are reminded that some reactions (e.g. the development of cancers, chloroquine retinopathy and retroperitoneal fibrosis) may become manifest months or years after drug exposure. Please report any suspicion of such an association.

2.   Drugs in the elderly. Doctors are asked to be particularly alert to the possibility of adverse reactions when drugs are given to the elderly.

3.   Congenital abnormalities. When an infant is born with a congenital abnormality or there is a malformed aborted foetus, doctors are asked to consider the possibility that this might be an adverse reaction to a drug and to report all drugs (including self-medication) taken by the mother during pregnancy.

4.   Vaccines. Doctors are asked to report all suspected reactions to both new and established vaccines. The balance between risks and benefits from vaccines is liable to change and needs to be kept under constant review.

As far as data sheets are concerned, the Medicines (Data Sheet) Regulations 1972 cover these, the relevant part being Schedule 2, Regulation 3(1), paragraph 5:

"Contra-indications, Warnings, etc.

5.   Contra-indications, warnings, precautions and action to be taken in the event of overdosage, relating to the medicinal product and main side effects and adverse reactions likely to be associated therewith and, where there are no such particulars to be given, a statement to that effect shall be made; where required in the interests of safety, the antidote or other appropriate action to be taken".

It is to be noted that it refers to main side effects and adverse reactions. Unlike the U.S.A. regulations, the terms are not defined and are, therefore, open to different interpretations.

These then are the regulations covering marketed drugs, i.e. those with a product licence.

UNITED STATES OF AMERICA

The requirements in the U.S.A. are the strictest and most exact of any country as far as adverse reactions are concerned. The laws are laid out in the Federal Register by the Department of Health and Human Services through the Food and Drug Administration (F.D.A.).   When investigations in humans are about to start, a submission must be made for a Notice of Claimed Investigational Exemption for a New Drug (IND). The investigations carried out under the IND will result (one hopes) in a New Drug Application (NDA) on form 356H.   In Phase 3 and 4 of the clinical studies adverse drug experiences are reported to the F.D.A. by means of a simple form - the FDA 1639 (manufacturers) and FDA 1639(a) (clinicians).   Practising physicians are not obliged by law to notify the F.D.A. of adverse drug experiences but are requested to do so.   Investigations may continue under an IND long after an NDA has been approved. At the time of the benoxaprofen problem the regulations did not specifically require updating of the NDA after it was submitted although periodic reports were required to the IND.   Dr. R. Temple, Director of the Office of New Drug Evaluations, then asked for submission of all case reports involving a death or drug discontinuation because of an adverse event to the NDA and not the IND.   Changes in the regulations concerning the IND and NDA are imminent but in the meantime the 1977 regulations remain in force.   The latter are outlined first, followed by extracts from the proposed new regulations.   Regulations are frequently interpreted by official guidelines from the F.D.A.   Comments on this subject from the American Pharmaceutical Manufacturers' Association (P.M.A.) are often invaluable.

Pre-marketing

Investigational Exemption for a New Drug (IND)

After a drug has been fully researched in animals it is possible to apply for Investigational Exemption for a New Drug under the Code of Federal Regulations, Title 21, Chapter 1, Part 312, Sub-part A, Section 312-1, Subsection 2.

Paragraph 6. "With the application there must be a statement covering all information available to the sponsor derived from pre-clinical and any clinical studies and experience with the drug."

Paragraph 7. "It must also include an accurate description of the prior investigations and experiences and their results pertinent to the safety and possible usefulness of the drug........... It shall not represent that the safety or usefulness of the drug has been established for the purposes to be investigated. It shall describe all relevant hazards, contraindications, side effects and precautions suggested by prior investigation and experience with the drug................."

Paragraph 10 requires details of planned investigations within the U.S.A., states that the investigators must make a full statement of any adverse effects and useful results observed, together with an opinion as to whether such effects or results are attributable to the drug under investigation.

Subsection 5 requires that "accurate progress reports" must be made "at reasonable intervals not exceeding one year".

Subsection 6 requires that the "sponsor shall promptly investigate and report to the F.D.A. and all investigators any findings associated with the use of the drug that may suggest significant hazards, contraindications, side effects and precautions pertinent to the safety of the drug. If the finding is alarming it shall be reported immediately."

Subsection 7. "If the investigations adduce facts showing that there is substantial doubt that they may be continued safely in relation to the drug's potential therapeutic effects, the sponsor shall promptly discontinue the investigation...................."

Subsection 13 requires each investigator to fill in an FD 1573 which in paragraph 4(d) states "Any adverse effects that may reasonably be regarded as caused by or probably caused by the new drug shall be reported to the sponsor promptly..................."

New Drug Application (NDA)

The F.D.A. requirements for a New Drug Application are set out in the Code of Federal Regulations, Title 21, Chapter 1, Part 314, New Drug Applications, No. 187, September 27th 1977, subpart A, section 1. The relevant paragraphs are:

314.1.C.3.b. which says that the Application for a New Drug (NDA) should:

> "Include tabulation of all side effects or adverse experiences by age, sex and dosage formulation, whether or not considered to be significant, showing whether administration of the drug was stopped and showing the investigator's name with a reference to the volume and page number in the application.............. Indicate those side effects or adverse experiences considered to be drug related."

314.1.C.12.c.

"and a full statement of adverse effects and useful results observed, together with an opinion as to whether such effects are attributable to the drug under investigation."

314.1.C.12.d.

"Attach ...... a completed Form FD 1639 ...... for each adverse experience or, if feasible, for each subject or patient experiencing one or more adverse effects described in item 12c."

314.1.C.12.e.

"All information pertinent to an evaluation of the safety and effectiveness of the drug received or otherwise obtained by the applicant from any source including information derived from other investigations or commercial marketing (for example outside the United States) or reports in the scientific literature involving the drug that is the subject of the application and related drugs."

Postmarketing

As far as drugs once they are on the market are concerned, these are covered by the Code of Federal Regulations, Title 21, Chapter 1, Part 310, section 300, subpart D. Antibiotics are covered by Part 431, section 60.

310:300

(a) "...... the applicant shall establish and maintain records and make reports ...... including adequately organised and indexed files containing full reports of any of the following kinds of information pertinent to the safety or effectiveness of the drug.

   (1) Unpublished reports of clinical experience, studies, investigations and tests conducted by the applicant or reported to him by any person involving the drug and related drugs.

   (6) Information concerning the quantity of the drug distributed in a manner and form that facilitates estimates of the incidence of any adverse effects reported to be associated with the drug.

   (7)(b) The applicant shall submit to the F.D.A. ...... including   Forms FD 1639.

   (7)(b) (2) As soon as possible and in any event within 15 working days of its receipt by the applicant complete records or reports concerning drug information of the following kinds:

      (1) Information concerning any unexpected side effect, injury, toxicity or sensitivity reaction of any unexpected inci-

dence or severity thereof associated with clinical uses, studies and investigations or tests, whether or not determined to be attributable to the drug. "Unexpected" .... refers to conditions or developments not previously submitted as part of the NDA or not encountered during clinical trials of the drug or conditions or developments occurring at a rate higher than shown by information previously submitted as part of the request for certification or than encountered during clinical trials. In order to achieve reasonable uniformity in evaluating drug experience reports, the Division of Drug Experience (DDE) has had to establish a standard for measuring the "unexpected". The current product label was chosen as the standard, specific events/reactions listed in the warning, contraindication, adverse reaction, drug interaction, or laboratory interaction sections. Any event/reaction not listed in one of these sections is considered unexpected. Furthermore, any event which, although symptomatically and pathophysiologically related to a labelled event but which is not the same due to either greater severity, specificity or a variant, should be considered unexpected. For example, hepatic necrosis would be considered unexpected under this definition even if elevated hepatic enzymes or hepatitis were already noted in the label. Similarly, subarachnoid haemorrhage, cerebral thromboembolism or cerebral vasculitis would be considered unexpected if the label only referred to the occurrence of cerebral vascular accidents."

The draft guidelines for the use of FD 1639, page 5, also says:

"While only unexpected drug experiences technically fall under the 15-day requirement, DDE requests that serious known, serious rare, and fatal events also be reported within 15 days.

Severe/serious event is any event associated with a drug which is: 1) life threatening, 2) permanently disabling, 3) requires hospitalisation, 4) requires systemic drug or other therapy for treatment, or 5) is sufficiently incapacitating that the patient is unable to work or do usual activity. In addition, the following events are always considered severe/serious: death, congenital anomalies, cancer, overdoses, and lack of expected pharmacological effect.

Severe/serious is a term which DDE utilises to aid in the review and evaluation of ADR reports. Since the evaluation by DDE of a report for seriousness is independent of the evaluation for causality and "unexpectedness", this term can apply to both known and unexpected events."

"(7)(b) (4) All the information ...... shall be submitted at the following intervals ......

(1)   ...... within intervals of 3 months during the first year, within intervals of 6 months during the second year and at yearly intervals thereafter.

Section 301: Reporting (a) adverse drug experiences

(a)   (1)   All adverse experiences ...... shall also be reported on Form FD 1639

(2)   It is unnecessary for FD 1639 to be used in:-

(i)   Report ...... in Phase 1 and Phase 2.

(ii)   Submitted for adverse reactions reported in the published scientific literature.

(3)(b) ...... the terms "drug experience", "adverse drug experience" and "adverse reaction" mean any adverse experience associated with the use of the drug whether or not considered drug related and include any side effect, injury, toxicity or sensitivity reaction or significant failure of expected pharmacological action."

Subpart C : Records and Reports

Section 431:60 gives the records and reports concerning experience with antibiotic drugs for human use and is essentially similar to section 310:300 as far as adverse reactions are concerned.

This then is the gist of the regulations. Interpretation of these regulations is provided in F.D.A. Guidelines relevant to the various groups of drugs.

In 1981 the American Pharmaceutical Manufactuers' Association (P.M.A.) produced a New Drug Application Format Manual "to encourage conformity of the regulations and consistency in presentation". Pages 20 to 28 are essential reading since they describe how laboratory data and adverse reaction data should be laid out. The address of the P.M.A. is 1100 Fifteenth Street, N.W., Washington D.C. 2005, Area Code 202 835 3540.

The present situation (December 1983)

The F.D.A. has proposed to revise the New Drug Application regulation 47 Fed. Reg. 46627 (Oct 19 1982) and in December 1982 produced a draft guideline for the use of FD 1639 "Drug Experience Report". The important ADR changes in the proposed revision of the IND and NDA regulations are as follows:

IND Rewrite (June 1983)

ADR reports from IND trials will have to be reported within 3 working days if they concern fatal or life-threatening clinical experiences associated with the use of the drug not previously reported, i.e. where there is a reasonable possibility that the event may have been caused by the drug. Any other serious adverse experience associated with the drug, not previously reported, that may suggest significant hazards, contraindications, side effects or precautions will be notified as soon as possible and in no event later than 10 working days after the sponsor received the information. Sponsors will need to report follow-up information to both the 3 and 10 working day reports as "expeditiously as practicable" in an information amendment. This proposal covers all information relevant to the safety of the drug from any source, foreign or domestic, and includes clinical investigations, commercial marketing experience and published and unpublished papers.

NDA Rewrite

The term "adverse drug experience" has a proposed new definition: "any experience associated with the use of a drug in humans whether or not considered drug related" and this would include:

(1)   all suspected ADR

(2)   reactions occurring from drug overdose whether accidental or intentional

(3)   reactions occurring from drug abuse

(4)   reactions occurring from drug withdrawal

(5)   the failure of a drug's expected pharmacological action.

The F.D.A. would require all fatal and life-threatening adverse drug experiences that are not mentioned in the drug's current labelling to be notified within 15 working days. This would be called an "alert report". All other adverse drug experiences would have to be notified within 30 working days.

Other proposed changes include permitting an applicant to use any format for computer generated reports subject to the approval of the FDA Division of Drug Experience. Also reports of adverse drug experience reported in published literature need only to be reported to the F.D.A. if they involve adverse drug events or clinical toxicity information and these reports to the F.D.A. will be accompanied by a copy of the original publication as well as form FD 1639.

The new regulations will require an update to the NDA every four months and following the receipt of an approvable letter. These safety update reports will be similar in format to the original application and will be required until the approval letter is received and then annual reports will be required.

FRANCE

Premarketing

According to Article L601 of the Code de la Santé Publique there are three stages in premarketing studies:

1.   The analytical stage concerning the basic chemical, intermediate compounds and final product.

2.   The toxicological and pharmacological stage in animals.

3.   The clinical stage concerning efficacy and possible side effects in man.

Careful observation both for efficacy and for possible side effects must be undertaken simultaneously such that one can define precisely the conditions in which the medication should be used in current practice if the "autorisation de mise sur la marché" (A.M.M.) is given.   The A.M.M. is equivalent to a product licence.

Each phase is undertaken by an expert chosen from a list supplied by the Ministry of Health (Article R5120).   Each patient's results must be recorded in detail on the trial record form.   The form should contain all the information such that one can appreciate the beneficial effects and the tolerance of the medication (Journal Officiel 11.1.1975).

In Chapter II paragraph 12 of the Journal Officiel mentioned above (Protocol applicable a l'expertise clinique du medicament) concerning the clinical information on individual patients which is to be reported from the pre-marketing clinical trials, it states "all information on the reported side effects, noxious or not, as well as the measures taken in consequence of it: the cause-effect relationship must be studied with the same care as that which one applies normally to the identification of a therapeutic effect".

Postmarketing

In 1973 a National Centre for Pharmaceutical Surveillance was set up in France.   This was subsequently modified by decree on the 30th July 1982. The result was that there are:

(1)   Regional pharmaceutical surveillance (pharmacovigilance) centres, 28 in all, scattered across France.   Amongst other duties, they compile information about all serious incidents that could be related to the use of pharmaceutical products and about all incidents or accidents where a relationship between the use of products and the effects is thought possible.

(2)   A technical committee co-ordinates the collection of information from the regional centres as well as co-ordinating their other work.

This committee then passes all the information so collected to the National Commission of Pharmacovigilance.

(3)   The National Commission for Pharmacovigilance evaluates the validity of the data gathered and undertakes any necessary checking and monitoring. It also receives information directly from the pharmaceutical manufacturers, doctors, pharmacists and treatment centres for poisoning. As a result of this it may advise the Minister of Health of its findings.

A prescribing doctor may inform either the local pharmacovigilance centre directly, or via his own professional association, or the manufacturers by a yellow or green card system. The Syndicat National de l'Industrie Pharmaceutique (S.N.I.P.) advises the industry on the internal procedures to be followed with incoming information. S.N.I.P. state: "In France according to existing regulations the producer's responsibility in the field of pharmaceutical surveillance is limited to the statement of new effects that could endanger public health or modify the existing reports. That statement has to be made as soon as there is certainty and this implies that an enquiry has been made to check the existence of a causal effect between the administration of a product and the resulting effect". The working group of S.N.I.P. suggests that the manufacturers notify the technical committee periodically, or immediately if serious cases are involved, of all individually validated cases, whether they are known or not, should the causal effect be plausible or probable[116].

S.N.I.P. sent Circular No. 9974 on "Charter de Pharmacovigilance" on 15th September 1983 to all manufacturers. Included in the circular was advice on the notification of side effects. The latter are divided into:

1.   Older drugs, and
2.   Recently marketed drugs.

1.   **Older drugs**

All the facts which have been collected should be recorded in a chronological register for each product. Only unexpected or serious side effects need to be made the object of detailed enquiry and in the latter case the spontaneous notification can suffice as long as there is improved notification by the medical profession and the industry.

2.   **Recently marketed products**

Surveillance can be organised by structured studies either initiated by the manufacturer or requested by the administrative authorities or in liaison with them. Because of the problems inherent in structured studies, it is reasonable to limit them to drugs where special surveillance is indicated because of problems with existing drugs or because of problems found during premarketing studies. It is important that the manufacturer does not work in isolation but in liaison with regional and national organisations. The manufacturer must inform the authorities of serious cases or those where their use should be modified.

The law known as "Loi Talon" dated 7th July 1980 [Law No. 80-512 completing article L605 of the "Code de la Santé Publique] as paragraph 10 [Art. L605] details "the regulations applying to pharmaceutical surveillance as enforced on drugs after granting of the authorisation for marketing by the official authority", thereby establishing that the rules applied to drugs after authorisation to market the drug.

At the moment there is no obligatory declaration of side effects to the Ministry of Health either by the prescriber or the manufacturer. However, Article L601 of the Code of Public Health states that authorisation to market a drug does not exonerate the manufacturer or, where it is different, the holder of the authorisation, from the responsibility that one or the other has under common law by reason of the manufacturing or marketing of the product. Professor Dangoumau, who is now the head of the Direction de la Pharmacie et du Médicament, intends to put the whole system on a more sure footing. His previous post as Head of Pharmacovigilance at Bordeaux puts him in a very good position to improve the present situation.

Since there are currently no regulations governing a drug once it is on the market, requests from the government for the company to initiate some special form of surveillance can be, and often have been, ignored[263]. However, the authorisation for marketing is only for a period of five years. The renewal of this authorisation requires modification in the light of events whilst on the market.

Change in Regulation

Decree No. 84-402. Journal officiel 24 May 1984.
Article R 5144-8
All doctors, dentists and midwives having established an unexpected toxic effect which is possibly due to a drug they have prescribed must immediately inform the regional centre of Pharmacovigilance.

Article R 5144-9
All product licence holders must declare to the Commission National de la Pharmacovigilance all unexpected toxic effects which are possibly due to the drug and of which they have knowledge. This should be done every 3 months for the first year and then annually.

WEST GERMANY

The law in West Germany governing the reporting of adverse drug reactions is the Medicines Act 1976 sometimes referred to as the AMG (Arznei-mittelgesetz).

Premarketing

The registration documents which must be submitted to the authority in order to get approval to market a new drug are dealt with under Sections 22-24. The reporting of "side effects" is dealt with under Section 22, paragraph 1, No. 8, and "results of the clinical testing" under Section 22, paragraph 2, No. 3. These specify that any adverse events noted must be listed as follows:

> "Please specify the unwanted symptoms observed and state the frequency of occurrence of each symptom. The list should start with the most frequent symptom and end with the least frequent. For each symptom please state the shortest and the longest time interval between the beginning of the therapy being tested and the first occurrence of the symptoms in question. State the number of patients in whom the adverse effects were observed. If dose-dependent occurrence of a side effect was observed, advise accordingly. Describe briefly what measures against adverse effects were effective or might be supposed to have been effective. Detail the consequences of use not in accordance with directions, and their treatment, if observations in this connection are available. Finally, give an opinion on the question of psychical and physical dependence."

Once the registration documents have been submitted to the Bundesgesundheitsamtes (B.G.A.) any changes with regard to side effects must immediately be notified by the company according to Section 29 (pre- and post- marketing).

Postmarketing

Section 49, paragraph 6 of the Medicines Act states:

> "The pharmaceutical concern is under an obligation to submit to the competent Federal authority a report of experience gained with a medicine which contains a substance or a preparation as referred to in Para. 4 No. 1 after a period of two years from the specification of the substance issued under Section 4, No. 1. The report must contain information about the quantities issued in the period, any new information about effects, the type and frequency of side effects, contraindications, interactions with other agents, any habituation, any dependency or any inappropriate use must be detailed."

The references to "a medicine which contains a substance or a preparation as referred to in Para. 4, No. 1" refers to new chemical entities which come under "prescription only" regulations for the first five years following submission. This "report of experience" should be completed in accordance with the following directions:

3.   If the substance is contained in several presentations and strengths a separate report has to be submitted for each of these products......

5.   ...... We ask you to estimate how many patients have been treated with the product based on a mean dosage and a mean duration of treatment.

6.   ...... Please summarise the number of adverse events reported following administration of the product. These should be specified according to the type of adverse event. Please state which of these reports, to your knowledge, have already been submitted to the B.G.A. or A.M.K. in order to avoid the cases being registered twice.

The summary of adverse events should contain a statement in which cases the company supposes a causal relationship between the administration of the drug and the adverse event reported to be certain, probable, possible, unlikely or not clear.

7.   If available, please give further details, e.g. diagnosis, daily dose, duration of administration, which are relevant for an appropriate evaluation......

8.   Please summarise your knowledge on the use in practice of your product and give an evaluation......

Please state also which measures concerning the safety of drugs you have taken according to new information on the drug (e.g. addition of warnings of adverse events which were not known at the time of registration) and which legal measures you think appropriate (e.g. release from the automatic prescription only regulations).

9.   The knowledge about benefits and risks of medical products are not limited to borders. If a drug is also used abroad, please include the experience gained in other countries in your report. This should be compiled in an extra documentation.

Please state in which countries the drug was approved since the product licence was granted in West Germany. Please state which indications and which side effects are registered in these countries; please state also if it is available on prescription only.

Section 62 requires that the Federal Authority collects centrally and evaluates information relating to side effects, interactions with other agents, contraindications and any adulterations. Liaison with the World Health Organisation (W.H.O.), the medicine authorities of other countries and various internal bodies recording risks from medicines is also one of the authority's functions.

The pharmaceutical companies are obliged to report side effects to the Arzneimittelkommission der Deutschen Ärzteschaft (A.M.K.) (an independant body of 36 clinicians within the German Medical Council) and also to the B.G.A. The latter evaluate the reports which are then discussed at meetings which are held at regular intervals.

Dr. Ochsenfahrt of the Medicines Commission of the West German medical profession has proposed four measures for improving the collection of adverse reactions in West Germany:

1. Substituting early and complete information exchange between doctors, manufacturers and authorities for the present process;

2. Intensification of the medical profession's reporting of side effects;

3. Manufacturers to make more use of specific prospective monitoring of approved substances;

4. All products should have the date of their approval clearly stated on the pack, or be labelled with a symbol for two to four years after approval. The doctors would then be asked to be aware of this symbol and to report all adverse reactions occurring during treatment.

The standard references to the arzneimittelgesetz in Germany are:-

1. AMG (Arzneimittelgesetz)
   Gesetz zur Neuordnung des Arzneimittelrechtes of 24 August 1976 published in the Bundesgesetzblatt Page 2445, 2448. Changes in the law were announced in the Bundesgesetzblatt from 24 Feb.1983 Vol 1 page 169.

2. Arzneimittelrecht
   Kommentar fuer die juritische und pharmazeutische Praxis zum neuen Gesetz neben den Verkehr mit Azneimitteln. (Arzneimittelgesetz) by Sander A, Koebner H.E., Scholl H.O. Publisher Verlag W. Kohlhammer GmbH, Koeln, Stuttgart, Berlin, Mainz 1977/1983.

This book is an essential commentary to the interpretation of the AMG.

ITALY

Pre-marketing

Circular No. 54bis : 30.3.1967

If a drug has been registered and on sale in another country for two years, a special report, giving all the beneficial effects and all the secondary effects of this usage and of the extensive trials undertaken there in man, must be compiled, translated and certified. Under these circumstances only minimal research may be necessary in Italy.

Circular No. 77 : 6.9.1975 – 800/2/AG351/6895

Clinical Trials

Clinical trials must establish possible side effects. They must report clinical results either favourable or unfavourable. All information collected regarding side-effects, either favourable or not and the steps taken to prevent the latter, must be reported. The drug relationship or causality must be studied with the same effort as the search for therapeutic activity. All information regarding general tolerability and information regarding laboratory tests that have been performed before and after treatment, distinguishing the effect deriving from the drug and from the excipient. A conclusion must be given regarding each observed event.

Postmarketing

The drug company is required to submit to the board of the Pharmaceutical Service of the Ministry of Health information reports on each drug at prescribed intervals, which are six-monthly for the first two years and then annually for a further three years. The report should contain:

1. details of the number of packs produced and sold and an estimate of the number of patients who have taken the drug.

2. details of the nature and frequency of any toxic or secondary effects, either local or generalised, as may be consequent upon or in any way related to the use of the drug and which may have come to the notice of the company in any way whatsoever.

3. documentation of all the side effects reported in any clinical trial concerning the drug undertaken subsequent to marketing and published anywhere in the world.

(Ref. Articles 1 and 2, Ministerial Decree 20.3.1980, Official Gazette of the Italian Republic No. 83).

Article 8 – Ministerial Decree No. 480 – 2.7.1981

When a doctor has observed a toxic secondary effect or unexpected result from a drug, either a localised or generalised reaction deriving or in any way linked with the use of the drug, then he must fill in the official form. He may send a copy to the Health Ministry but the pharmaceutical company must collect the form, if necessary using their representatives for this purpose.

Circular No. 106 : 15.12.1975 - 800/1/AG2/5/54/9992

Data Sheet

The data sheet must contain what has been observed by the use of the drug. It must agree entirely with the data sheet of the country which performed the basic research. An official translation of any other data sheets from the first country that registered the drug and any subsequent countries must be submitted.

JAPAN

Pre-marketing

The reporting system of ADR prior to approval in Japan, including the reporting of the ADR found in foreign countries, consists of the following two types:

1.   Submission of a list of adverse drug events as a part of the New Drug Application (NDA) data.

2.   Reporting of adverse events during studies in the registration work.

All the adverse events other than those to be reported during the registration work must be included in the list to be submitted at the time of the NDA.

The reporting system of ADR prior to approval is not stipulated in regulations but instructions are given for administrative guidance:

1.   A list of adverse reactions to be submitted to the Ministry of Health and Welfare (MHW) as a part of the NDA data.

      This is required in order to show the grounds for "Precautions for use" in "Data concerning the results of clinical trials" to be included in the NDA data. The points requiring special attention are:

      (a)   All adverse reactions observed in all trials carried out in Japan must be tabulated into:

             (i)   A list of adverse events.

             (ii)   A list of abnormal laboratory findings

             Detailed information on the symptoms and the course of the adverse events must be provided, together with the comments by the doctor in charge, including his views on the reversibility of the symptoms on drug withdrawal, etc.

      (b)   The incidence of adverse events must be stated for double-blind comparative studies and for open clinical trials respectively and, if there is a difference in the incidence between the double-blind studies and the open clinical trials, the difference must also be explained.

(c)   For serious adverse events, such as death, including those in foreign data, detailed information of the case, causal relationship, etc., must be provided.

(d)   There is no stipulation on reporting of the adverse events reported only in overseas countries (e.g. those stated in data sheets or physicians' reference material), but serious or special (unusual) reactions or those on which the authorities require information must be submitted to the MHW, i.e. the relevant published papers and also such information must be reflected in the "Precautions for use" in the package leaflet in Japan.

2.   Report of adverse drug events found during registration work.

Any information which is very important concerning the efficacy or safety of a drug under investigation, e.g. that clinical trials were discontinued because of the occurrence of harmful adverse reactions, must be reported to the MHW.   There is no fixed format for such reporting but it is recommended that an appropriate format would be similar to that used in postmarketing adverse event reports.

JAPAN

Postmarketing

This can be divided into two parts:

1.   Regular annual reports.

2.   Voluntary reporting system.

Regular annual reports

Drugs are allowed on to the Japanese market subject to re-examination over either a four or six year period. It is six years for drugs which have new active ingredients not previously approved (includes combined drugs with active ingredients or compositions different from those of the combined drugs previously approved) and drugs where the route of administration is new but the active ingredients are already approved. It is four years where the active ingredients and route of administration have already been approved but where the indications and effects are apparently different or where the administration and dose are apparently different. When a new drug with the same active ingredients, administration and dosage, and indications and effects as those of an already approved drug is approved during the re-examination period of the already approved drug, the re-examination period for the new drug is the remainder of the re-examination period for the already approved drug.

The re-examination period (i.e. four or six years) must cover at least 10,000 patients and reports are required yearly as to its progress. The first three years are spent on collecting the data on the 10,000 patients and the remaining period for other special investigations. In the plan submitted by the manufacturer before approval for the carrying out of this task reference has to be made to:

(a) Problems regarding safety at the time of the development of the drug.

(b) Problems regarding safety with similar drugs.

(c) Problems regarding safety resulting from the experience in foreign countries.

This plan must contain a copy of the adverse reaction investigation card and a list of the incidence of adverse reactions so far discovered.

The plan for these investigations is accepted, for each drug, by the Ministry of Health and Welfare (MHW) but obviously amongst the requirements are investigations concerning adverse reactions and general safety of the drug. These latter are considered under the following points:

(a) Items related to the actual incidence of adverse reactions (types, degree, frequency, etc.), efficacy and conditions of use (directions and dose, period of use, reason for use, reason for withdrawal, etc.), conditions concerning patients (age, sex, complications, medical histories, constitutions, etc.), drugs and methods of treatment used concomitantly, etc.

(b) The degree of the symptoms, period required for improvement, preventative measures, treatment methods, etc., in the case of adverse reactions which require special precautions (e.g. eye or ear disorders, muscular or skeletal disorders, nervous disorders, blood disorders, organ dysfunctions, etc.).

(c) Items concerning adverse reactions and efficacy not known at the time of approval:

e.g. delayed adverse reactions, adverse reactions and effects appearing during long-term continuous use, use in suckling infants, small children, the elderly, pregnant women, etc.

(d) Research reports concerning the safety and efficacy of the new drug concerned:

e.g. case reports, epidemiological survey reports, results of animal experiments, physiochemical test results, etc., appearing in domestic or foreign scientific journals or in the reports of research performed by the manufacturing company itself or related companies.

The incidence of adverse reactions by type and the results of analysis of the adverse reaction incidence must be reported yearly.

(Ref. Notice from Director-General of Pharmaceutical Affairs Bureau Yakuhatsu No. 483 issued on 10.4.1980, 4 of Article 21 of Enforcement Regulations of Pharmaceutical Affairs Law, 2-4 of Article 14 of the revised Pharmaceutical Affairs Law).

Voluntary reporting system

Information on adverse reactions should be actively and carefully collected and their reporting to the MHW is obligatory and should be done within 30 days (if further investigation is still required, the reason for this delay must be given).

Adverse reactions to be reported include:

(a)   Adverse reaction thought to be caused by the drug but which are not mentioned in the precautions for use.

(b)   Serious adverse reactions (those which caused death or disability, those which might result in death or disability, and those which are found to be severe by the physician in charge among the cases where recovery is difficult, etc.).

Any research report showing that serious adverse reactions, such as cancer, might occur, that the adverse reaction tendencies, such as the number of adverse reaction cases, incidence and onset conditions, have markedly changed or that the drug does not have the approved indications and effects.

(Ref. Notice from Director-General of Pharmaceutical Affairs Bureau Yakuhatsu No. 483 issued on 10.4.1980, 2 of Article 62 of Enforcement Regulations of Pharmaceutical Affairs Law, Article 69 of the revised Pharmaceutical Affairs Law).

The adverse reactions to be reported were given in more detail in a further notice (Yakuhatsu No. 298) on 27th April 1984.

(b) 'Disability' was defined as disablement, being the occurrence of such permanent dysfunction as to cause disturbance in daily life. 'Might result in death or disability' as a case indicating a possibility of resulting in death or such permanent dysfunction as to cause disturbances in daily life depending on the patient's physical disposition or conditions at the time of the occurrence of the adverse event.

'Those which are found to be severe' as showing such severity as to require hospitalization or attending a hospital for a considerable time and which the doctor or dentist in charge has judged as severe.

To a 'serious adverse reaction' has had added 'congenital abnormalities, sensory disorders and haematological disorders or research reports on occurrences or possibility of occurrence of such adverse events as circulatory failure, dermal disorders and organ disorders with the severity as defined above'.

This report also emphasizes the efforts needed by pharmaceutical companies to collect and report adverse events as follows:-

1.   Even if it is difficult to judge whether a case falls under the category requiring report or not, such a case should be reported.

2.   Pharmaceutical companies should review their system of collection and evaluation of information on adverse events and reinforce it for prompt and exact collection of such information. Also they should evaluate the collected information before reporting to the authorities.

3.   The companies associated with overseas companies should endeavour to collect actively adverse event data from their overseas associated companies.

8

The Collection, Storage, Retrieval and Management of Adverse Drug Reaction Data
(Guest Contributor: Dr J.C.C. Talbot)

INTRODUCTION

Several aspects of the handling of adverse drug reaction (ADR) data are discussed in this chapter, including the sources of data, form design, computerisation and analysis of data and codes for adverse events, diseases and drugs. The published literature on ADRs is also critically evaluated and the limitations of some literature searching methods are identified. Computer systems are discussed from the user's view.

The content reflects the author's personal experience. It is not meant to be a comprehensive review of the subject and in certain areas references only will be cited rather than reproducing their content. In practice each pharmaceutical company or regulatory authority has set up its own procedures and documentation to meet its exact needs and preferences. Hence, discussion will mainly be concerned with the broad objectives and principles; exact details are best left to individual choice.

SOURCES OF ADR DATA

Data on ADRs or adverse events can be derived from several different sources and there can be an enormous variation in nature and quality depending on the source. Before such data can be processed or computerised, two fundamental points must be considered. Firstly, to a large extent, the form and quality of the data dictates how it is to be handled and hence more than one method may be appropriate. Secondly, procedures and systems design must reflect the requirements for output which are, of course, also dictated by the first consideration. Data may come from any of the following sources:

Clinical trials	-	Phase 1 (volunteer studies)
	-	Phases 2 and 3 (premarketing trials)
	-	Phase 4 (post-marketing trials)
Spontaneous reports	-	Own country

	–	Overseas countries
	–	Regulatory Authority reports
Literature	–	Own country
	–	Overseas countries

Clinical trials

In Phase 1 studies good documentation and additional investigations should be possible but serious reactions are, fortunately, very unusual in these studies and rare reactions will not be detected due to the numbers involved. Good documentation and follow-up should be possible in Phase 2 and 3 studies but, again, rare reactions are unlikely to be identified. Phase 4 studies are often commercially rather than scientifically orientated and, although the larger numbers of patients involved may aid the detection of rare reactions, the quality of ADR data may be poor due to study design.

Spontaneous reports

Spontaneous reports are the most effective means of identifying rare reactions, despite the under-reporting that exists. However, the quality of reports is often inadequate and only through good form design or, alternatively, by the use of field workers, can pharmaceutical companies or regulatory authorities achieve satisfactory documentation. There is also a variation in the quality of spontaneous reports from country to country; although reports from the U.K. and U.S.A. have been described as poor, they are good in comparison with others. Some do not have a regulatory authority reporting form for ADRs, i.e. most third-world countries, and others have a very basic form which is not very helpful, e.g. Italy.

Clinical trials and spontaneous reports are considered further in subsequent sections.

Literature

The publication of case reports in medical and scientific journals is an important primary source of information on ADRs. The quality of ADR reports in the published literature is notoriously variable and has been the subject of much criticism and correspondence. Recently some guidelines have been given to authors of case reports, see below, and some journals have raised their standards for acceptance of such articles. The quality of such reports has probably improved in recent years and should continue to do so. Nevertheless, the impact of published case reports can be great and their value should not be under-estimated.

For many drugs there are now a vast number of publications; for example, there are some 3,500 papers concerning salbutamol and over 10,000 concerning cimetidine. These quoted figures are for the total number of publications and include papers where the drug is only briefly mentioned and others dealing with chemical and analytical aspects as well as clinical work. However, a fairly high proportion are clinically orientated and some of these describe ADRs either in passing or in considerable detail. These large numbers of papers are spread throughout the ever-increasing number of scientific and biomedical journals now published. Conversely, for some drugs, particularly recently marketed compounds, there is a scarcity of clinical publications and frequently there is an inadequate account of the adverse reaction profile. Clearly, even for ADRs alone, it is only feasible for a practitioner to keep abreast with a limited number of journals, or papers on a very small group of drugs, hence the need for drug information specialists.

Dr Judith Jones, of the F.D.A., has recently proposed minimal information elements that are required to draw any conclusion about the possible relationship between a drug and an adverse event[264]. The criteria for these basic data elements in published reports are closely related to those for ADR causality assessment using algorithms or scoring lists (see Chapter 3) and are also a useful guide for anyone collecting data on ADRs. The following points, considered to be essential by Jones[264], can be adapted and developed for a potential checklist, as follows:

1.   **Timing**

   1.1   How long had the patient been receiving the suspected drug before the adverse event?

   1.2   What other drugs had been taken and for how long?

   1.3   Were there other relevant factors, e.g. diet, occupational exposure, etc.?

2.   **Dechallenge**

   2.1   Was the suspected drug stopped or continued?

   2.2   If stopped, did the adverse event disappear or improve?

   2.3   What was the time course of the above?

   2.4   Was the time course consistent with the drug's kinetics and the dynamics of the disease process?

3.   **Rechallenge**

   3.1   Was the patient rechallenged with the suspected drug?

   3.2   Did the adverse event recur in a reasonable time course?

4.   **Alternative causes**

   4.1   What other conditions or factors were present or possibly present that could have accounted for the adverse event?

5.   **Patient details**

   5.1   Age, sex, race, body weight, etc.

   5.2   Previous medical history.

Despite the anecdotal nature and sometimes poor documentation, publication of case reports in journals still remains one of the most useful primary sources of information on ADRs.   Journals should continue to publish such reports, although there is always the risk of false alarms. However, this problem is recognised; the British Medical Journal now "aims at steering a path between the extremes of crying wolf too often and insisting on near certain evidence"[184].

There are a number of excellent reference books on ADRs, notably the Meyler's Side Effects of Drugs series.   However, the problem with all of these books is the time-lag between a reaction being reported in the primary literature and its inclusion in the publication.   This is a particular problem with new drugs and newly reported reactions with established drugs.   It can largely be overcome in two ways; firstly by using abstracting services and, secondly, by "on-line" literature searching.   A number of abstracting publications are available, for example "Inpharma"   and "Reactions", both of which are published by ADIS Press, New Zealand. "Inpharma" is available weekly and has a short lag-time but only a small part has been devoted to ADRs since the introduction in January 1980 of "Reactions" which is available fortnightly and deals exclusively with ADRs. There is also "Clin-Alert" which also covers only ADRs and is published fortnightly by Science Editors Inc., Louisville, Kentucky, U.S.A., but appears to have a greater lag-time and is less useful in the author's experience.   All these abstracting services are valuable in providing fairly recent information from a wide range of journals but their cost probably confines them to specialist units.

On a similar note there is the National Abstracting Scheme which is a co-operative venture by hospital drug information pharmacists in the U.K. This was formally started in 1977 as a low cost scheme to meet the needs of drug information pharmacists[265], although it drew together a number of smaller schemes already in existence.   The Scheme had 23,500 papers key-worded and abstracted on microfiche at the end of 1983 and about 25% of these concerned, at least in part, ADRs.   Approximately 85 journals are scanned by the participating pharmacists[265], the choice of journals having changed considerably since the start of the scheme.   The time-lag between a paper appearing and being abstracted is about two weeks for the weekly core journals and a month or more for others.   Apart from the selected journals, C.S.M. publications, such as "Current Problems", and some D.H.S.S. circulars are also included.   The Scheme has provided a useful source of information and is now considerably more valuable as it is available on-line as "Pharmline".

"On-line" literature searching of commercially available databases, such as MEDLINE, EXCERPTA MEDICA and RINGDOC, has in recent years become available to many more users.   However, these facilities only partly overcome the time-lag, as it takes time for a paper to be indexed and incorporated in such databases. They are also not entirely comprehensive in journal coverage, particularly with conference abstracts and proceedings. In an examination of six databases for publications on cimetidine it was shown how some performed better in particular areas, e.g. pharmacological papers, clinical papers, abstracts or reviews, and that more than one database was needed to approach 100% recovery[266].

In the search for ADR reports on these databases two other problems are worthy of comment. Firstly, the indexers who compile the systems apply certain selection criteria to restrict the number of index terms used, and this may result in some drugs or adverse reactions not being indexed if they are a secondary part of the paper. For example, a paper describing reports received by the Australian Drug Reactions Advisory Committee[267] referred to many ADR reports, but the drugs and reactions were not indexed, hence the paper would not be identified by a search for any of the ADRs mentioned. Secondly, there is the problem of "false drops". If a search is conducted using the appropriate terms for the desired drug and adverse reaction, a list of papers will be obtained. However, in practice they do not all necessarily describe or refer to the drug causing the reaction because it is not possible to link directly the drug with the adverse reaction. This is because references to the drug being used in the treatment of a patient with that disease or reaction, and separate coincidental mentions in a paper will also be selected. This problem can be overcome by more sophisticated indexing techniques, such as relational indexing which is available with CAIRS[268], but as regards the drug literature these are only currently employed within the pharmaceutical industry.

Pharmaceutical companies and other specialists, such as drug information pharmacists need, therefore, to establish their own literature systems for the following reasons:

1.   Journal coverage requirements

2.   Decreased time-lag

3.   Special indexing and searching techniques to increase precision and avoid false drops

4.   Particular output requirements, such as abstracts and various formats

There are a number of commercially available software packages which are suitable for literature information systems, and in some cases for clinical trials and spontaneous reports as well e.g. CAIRS, STAIRS, ASSASSIN AND STATUS. However, before opting for one of these packages, the following points should be carefully considered:

1.   What are the applications and exact requirements of the planned system and how well does each package meet them?

2. What other applications does the package have and might it be shared with other user groups and thus spread the cost?

3. Does it work well on existing hardware?

4. How much space is occupied, i.e. does it affect other system users?

5. Is there a need for specialised computing support?

6. What after-sales service is available, i.e. software adaptations, training and further development?

7. Requirements for peripheral equipment (terminals/printers).

8. Interface with existing office equipment, e.g. wordprocessors.

9. Degree of user friendliness.

10. Degree of user control over software.

11. Problems in conversion of backlog data.

12. Who inputs data - validation and verification procedures, batch entry or on-line?

13. Who will do the indexing/abstracting?

14. Robustness of package.

15. Cost.

The purchase of such a package is a major undertaking and requires a high level of organisation and commitment throughout to be successful. A thesaurus is often considered necessary and offers many advantages but will involve a considerable amount of development. There is no such thing as an "ideal" thesaurus and everybody's requirements differ. Although MeSH (see later) may be a useful starting point, most users have developed their own.

Some systems designed primarily for literature are also suitable for spontaneous reports and even clinical trials, should the user want a combined system. With appropriate design, it is possible to search both published literature and spontaneous reports simultaneously to answer the perennial question "has such and such a reaction ever been reported with this drug".

ADR FORMS AND FORM DESIGN

A large number of different forms are used by different organisations for essentially the same purpose of collecting information about an ADR. Most Western regulatory authorities have their own form, see appendix for examples (CSM yellow card and FDA 1639) and, although the elements of these are similar, little attempt has been made to standardise the design. However, several countries do use the WHO reporting form to transmit data to the WHO research centre for international monitoring of adverse reactions to drugs[269]. Similarly, most pharmaceutical companies have their own such form, or forms, and not surprisingly collaboration to produce a standard design has been minimal.

Although the forms have the same purpose, the design must reflect their users' requirements. On one hand a regulatory authority probably wants to make reporting as simple as possible and is mainly concerned that the adverse event has occurred in association with a certain drug. Thus, a basic form is desirable. A pharmaceutical company, on the other hand, probably prefers far more data to help determine the causal relationship between the event and their product. Thus, the user must first define what data they wish to collect. The next step concerns what happens to the form once it is returned, i.e. data processing. Points such as whether the form is to serve as a direct entry document or whether there is need for a transcription document, must also be considered (see later).

When designing the form, all the usual factors in form and record design need to be considered, e.g. size, layout, colour, print, case, spacing, flow of questions, boxes, language and instructions. The main points in a series of articles [270-272] in the British Medical Journal on design of forms for clinical trials are also applicable to ADR form design. Another factor in ADR form design might be compatibility with other ADR forms, notably certain regulatory authority forms. The FDA, for instance, require ADR reports to be submitted on their Drug Experience Report Form (FDA 1639). Thus, if a pharmaceutical company does not want to use this form itself, but needs to submit reports to the FDA, it will need to design a form which is compatible.

A number of forms designed partly by the authors and used by the Glaxo Group of companies are also included in the appendix. 'Form 1' is considered as a general purpose reporting form, containing the basic elements of data to determine causality but not providing very much space for laboratory values. It is used for general practitioners, hospital cases where there is little laboratory data and for most overseas subsidiary companies. Form 1 is printed as a folding postage pre-paid envelope for UK use to further encourage a good response. 'Form 2' is for hospital reports where laboratory data and biopsy reports are relevant. The Skin Form is designed for the simple descriptive recording of adverse skin reactions and an earlier version proved useful in determining the nature of skin reactions with labetalol. These skin forms were designed in conjunction with Dr C. J. Stevenson, Consultant Dermatologist, Royal Victoria Infirmary, Newcastle upon Tyne. It is also envisaged that other specialised forms may be required, e.g. for anaesthetic drugs and for drug overdose (The Wellcome Foundation has a form for the latter[273]).

It will be noted that the design of the Glaxo forms is basically modular. Thus, a more sophisticated form can be built up from the simple one whilst preserving common data fields for computerisation, and selected modules can be used for other applications, such as clinical trial record forms. The basic modules of the Form 1 are:

1. Patient details

2. Relevant medical history

3. Drugs

4. Adverse event(s)

5. Treatment of adverse event

6. Laboratory data

7. Reporter

The form could easily be enlarged to accommodate a bigger laboratory data module and for clinical trials modules 1, 2, 3, 6 and 7 would probably not be needed on the adverse event page, as they appear elsewhere in the clinical record forms.

COMPUTERISATION OF ADR DATA

In this section computer input and storage of ADR data from clinical trials and spontaneous reports will be considered in more detail, data analysis and output are discussed later. Before deciding on how data is to be computerised, the sources of data must be identified, together with the types of searches and output required, i.e. the users must decide what they want from the system. If the requirement is to see quickly whether a reaction has been reported before, how many cases and where from, etc., a fairly simple system, possibly combined with a literature system is appropriate. However, a system may be required to process data from ADR forms of varying complexity to give a range of analyses, such as patient age ranges, time to onset of reactions, doses, etc.

In many situations there will also be major constraints on the choice of system because of computer hardware and software packages already available. Some software packages are designed to cope with free text, some have sophisticated thesaural capability, whilst with others coded systems only are available. Most pharmaceutical companies already have large computer systems, in which case there may be a choice of joining the corporate system or setting up a small dedicated system. In the former case the available hardware and software may not be ideal but there will probably be good support from a computing department and new software could be purchased or written. In the latter case, considerably more resources may be needed by a small department and a small dedicated system may not have the searching power and flexibility of a big computer. Decisions on which is preferable must be made by weighing up the particular needs and circumstances. There are, however, several examples of systems that have been successfully developed on large computer systems by pharmaceutical companies[122, 245, 273, 274].

A major consideration is how the data is to be entered on to the computer and subsequently edited and updated. The two basic methods available are batch entry by data preparation staff and screen formatted entry. In the former case, documents must be totally unambiguous and all codes, etc., added before being given to staff who enter the data from a series of flagged boxes. Before this can be done, all documents must be checked and, if necessary, coded by data monitoring staff. This approach is now generally adopted for clinical trials where there is a need to computerise large volumes of data quickly with minimal updating. For adverse events, particularly spontaneous reports, it is not so easy or acceptable to design forms suitable for direct computer entry and a transcription document may be necessary. A further problem is that there is often further follow-up information to be added. The transfer of data from an ADR form to a transcription document is time-consuming and prone to error, although the end product can be quickly entered by data preparation staff. An example of a transcription document used by the Wellcome Research Laboratories in the U.K. appears in the Appendix. One method of checking that batches of data have been entered correctly is double entry, i.e. the data is input twice and the computer checks that the files are identical. It is also possible to validate the data to some extent by having only certain allowed entries for each field, e.g. numeric or alphabetic only, or a certain numeric range.

In the case of screen formatted entry, the data monitoring aspects (i.e. checking and coding) and the data entry can be done by the same staff. Verification by double entry is probably not feasible in this situation and a manual checking of output is more practical, providing the volume of data is not too large. Screen formatted entry in some situations is more time-consuming and prone to errors but the choice between the two methods is dependent on the staff and resources actually available. There is also the possibility of entering data either way and it may be most practical to input the original data by batch entry but make amendments and updates by screen entry.

CODING SYSTEMS AND THESAURI FOR ADVERSE EVENTS AND DISEASES

Introduction

It is logical to deal with adverse events and diseases using one system because:

1.   ADRs frequently mimic spontaneously occurring diseases, hence the same diagnosis or symptom could appear as an adverse event or a disease.

2.   To identify new ADRs it is important not to separate a possible side effect from a disease.

3.   Two separate systems could lead to confusion.

Whether a coding system or a structured textual system (i.e. a thesaurus) is selected depends largely on the user's requirements - either can work perfectly well.

Free text based systems are much simpler as far as data inputting is concerned, but present serious disadvantages for retrieval, particularly in the field of adverse events/diseases, as so many synonyms and spelling variations can be encountered. Serial searching can be much slower with controlled language systems, unless very large, fast computers are available. A thesaurus-based system is more user-friendly, because it is textually based but this may present difficulties for the non-typist on searching. However, a thesaurus takes up a lot of computer storage space and each term alone can be very long, thus making the system cumbersome. Errors on inputting can be checked by a machine-held thesaurus and are easier to see.

Coding systems tend to be preferred by computing staff, because they take up less storage space. However, they have a number of disadvantages as far as the user is concerned. Generally they are less user-friendly and possibly more prone to errors at the input stage. The coding system must be structured carefully, since diseases do not fall naturally into a decimal system. If a term is only allowed one code, it can only be in one place in the hierarchy which can cause problems. For example, should "eye infections" be included in eye disorders or infections? Cross-referencing may, therefore, be necessary. If however, a coding system is selected it is essential that an automatic decode facility is available so that computer output is meaningful and not just a list of codes that have to be translated manually.

The possible requirements for a system are discussed below but, once one is chosen, a high degree of commitment is necessary. It is preferable not only to use the one system for adverse events and diseases but to use it throughout for clinical data, i.e. data from phase 1 studies right through to phase 4 studies and spontaneous reports.

Possible requirements of a coding system/thesaurus

A number of possible requirements for an adverse events and diseases coding system are listed but these are only a guide and the users must decide their own requirements. A shorter, more simple list may be adequate for many users.

1.   Acceptable to all users

2.   Comprehensive - able to code any terms that may be encountered (diseases, symptoms or adverse events)

3.   Specific - code available for the actual term

4.   Hierarchical - ability to search general as well as specific concepts, for instance all eye effects, all skin effects, etc.

5. Controlled terminology - synonyms controlled by same or very similar code

6. Easy and rapid to use - preferably from a simple coding book or printout

7. No ambiguity - of terms or codes

8. Preserves the exact term or description used by the clinician

9. Validation on input.

10. Codes should be as short as possible - accuracy and time factor.

The amount of computer space available and staff resources are also important considerations when choosing a system.

Available coding systems/thesauri suitable for adverse events and diseases

There is no such thing as an ideal coding system or thesaurus, the choice reflects user needs. Whether a system is to be used for literature, spontaneous reports, clinical trials or a combination of these will influence the selection. None of the systems reviewed below meets all the above requirements and, therefore, it may be necessary to modify one or even create a new system (see later). It may also be possible to use a coding system and text together i.e. coding the general concept and entering as text the terms used by the clinician. This review is not comprehensive and naturally reflects the author's personal experience. The systems considered are:-

> COSTART
> ICD-9
> MeSH
> OXMIS
> SNOMED
> WHO - adverse reaction terminology
> Modification of above systems
> Creation of own system

COSTART

COSTART[275] uses terse abbreviated phrases (maximum 24 characters) as coding symbols to describe diseases/adverse events. There are also body system codes and terms can be linked to more than one body system, where necessary. With appropriate hardware/software, coding symbols may be translated into full text and body system codes generated automatically. COSTART has been used by the F.D.A. but is currently under review and being modified.

Advantages: 1.   Specific terms and hierarchical structure.

               2.   Published system used by others (particularly phar-
                     maceutical companies in the U.S.A.).

Disadvantages: 1.   Not very specific unless used in conjunction
                     with text.

               2.   Precision of description sometimes lost when trans-
                     lated to coding symbol.

               3.   Coding symbols lengthy - requiring a lot of space
                     and predisposing to errors.

ICD-9

ICD-9 is a morbidity and mortality coding system developed by the
W.H.O.[276]. It is a highly structured system with a hierarchy based
primarily on body systems but with other major categories, e.g. infectious
and parasitic diseases. Discrete ranges of three digits incorporate a body
system, e.g. Diseases of the digestive system (520-579) and sub-classi-
fications within that system, e.g. Diseases of oral cavity, salivary glands
and jaws (520-529).   Each three digit code defines a more specific
classification, e.g. Disorders of tooth development and eruption
(520) and a fourth digit subdivides this, e.g. Mottled teeth (5203).
Further terms are frequently listed below such headings and are
thus included under the four digit code.

Advantages: 1.   Easy to find existing terms/codes - good index.

               2.   Comprehensive.

               3.   Published reference source used by others (but often
                     modified).

               4.   Good hierarchical structure.

               5.   W.H.O. centres can assist with problems encountered
                     in coding or classification.

Disadvantages: 1.   No control of synonyms.

               2.   Broad searches would need to include more than one
                     number range, e.g. body system and symptoms.
                     However, this can be overcome by creating a prefix.

There is also a clinical modification of ICD-9 called ICD.9.CM which
offers some advantages over the basic system.

MeSH (Medical Subject Headings)

MeSH[277] is the structured and controlled language authority list used by the National Library of Medicine for indexing bibliographic material in the MEDLARS database. The descriptors are grouped into 15 major categories, and within each category the terms may be further organised into subcategories.

The categories relevant here are:

A   Anatomical Terms
B   Organisms
C   Diseases
D   Chemicals and Drugs

The 23 subcategories of section C, for instance, include:

C1   Bacterial and fungal diseases
C4   Neoplasms
C8   Respiratory tract diseases
C14   Cardiovascular diseases
C21   Injury, occupational diseases, poisoning
C23   Symptoms and general pathology

Within each subcategory there is a hierarchical structuring and under each broad term there is a progressive narrowing of terms.

The hierarchy in a subcategory is expressed in a coded fashion, for example:

C8   Respiratory tract diseases
C8.127   Bronchial diseases
C8.127.108   Asthma
C8.127.108.110   Asthma, exercise-induced

The true hierarchical relationship is embodied in the numeric code. For each numeric code there is a controlled language equivalent which consists of a medical/scientific definition of the term, together with guidance notes on how and under what circumstances that particular term should be used; the notes include suggestions for related terms.

Advantages: 1.   Good hierarchical structure.

                2.   Published system used by others.

                3.   Easy to find existing terms.

Disadvantages: 1.   Poor for synonyms and certain terms, in particular symptoms.

                2.   Lengthy codes and terms.

MeSH is a good bibliographic thesaurus as it was designed for this function but it is poor for clinical trials. Adaptations in both areas are possible, in particular it is a good starting point for users designing their own bibliographic thesaurus.

OXMIS

Oxmis is a system designed in Oxford for primary medical care[278,279]. It is a hybrid based on ICD-8 with parts from other systems, notably OPCS surgical codes. The code has a maximum of nine characters but may be as few as three.   The first two characters of the code are a prefix indicating the derivation of the code; where ICD codes are used, there is no prefix. The next four characters are the core of the code but the full four are not always used. The final three characters are the suffix; codes currently may use none, one or two suffix characters.

Advantages: 1.   Easy to find code if there is one.

2.   Published system used by others.

3.   Structural system based on ICD-8.

4.   Central and assessable coding source - but possibly not to be relied on in the future.

Disadvantages: 1.   Fair number of terms not found in code book or printout, therefore not very comprehensive.

2.   Searching not straightforward - based on number ranges and several systems; requires detailed knowledge of ICD-8 and other systems used.

3.   Suffixes are used for both synonyms and code extensions of ICD - requires detailed knowledge of systems to do search and interpret output.

SNOMED (2nd edition)

SNOMED is a system developed by the College of American Pathologists[280-282]. It is a multi-concept system with fields for Topography (prime field), Morphology, Aetiology, Function, Diseases, Procedures and Occupations. Each term has a six character code except the Disease and Procedures fields which are five characters. Generally two fields are required to code a term accurately - sometimes this entails linking a function or morphology term with a Topography term, e.g. M40000 (inflammation) + 160000 (pharynx) = pharyngitis. In other cases the Topography term is added to facilitate searching, e.g. DX300 (glaucoma) + TXX000 (eye) ensures that glaucoma is retrieved when searching for eye effects. A third field may be added when more detail is required, for instance the aetiology field may be used if the cause of a problem is known, e.g. Streptococcus pneumoniae pneumonia = M40000 (inflammation), T28000 (lung), E2542 (Strep. pneumoniae).

Advantages: 1.   Very comprehensive - also possible to code unusual concepts by combining terms.

                 2.   Specific terms and hierarchical structure.

                 3.   Published and used by others - including pharmaceutical companies in the U.S.A. and some in the U.K.

                 4.   Coding courses run in the U.S.A.

Disadvantages: 1.   Complex to use.

                 2.   Possibility of arriving at different codes for the same term.

                 3.   Workload and error problems.

                 4.   Long codes, hence could take a lot of computer space.

WHO - Adverse Reaction Terminology

The WHO - Adverse Reaction Terminology[269,283] consists of Preferred Terms, the full text of which (maximum 33 characters) is stored; synonyms are called Included Terms but these always point back to the Preferred Term. There are thirty System-Organ Classes designated by a four digit code, e.g. skin and appendages disorders 0100 and vision disorders 0431. One or more of these classes are added to the Preferred Term, as appropriate. There are also High Level Terms which group together similar Preferred Terms, e.g. Convulsions is the High Level Term covering all the Preferred Terms describing different types of convulsions.

Advantages: 1.   Easy to find a code for a term which is either a Preferred or Included Term.

                 2.   Published system used by others (modified in some cases).

                 3.   Specific terms and hierarchical structure.

Disadvantages: 1.   Mainly covers diseases which are recognised as being ADRs, thus it is less suitable for event type data.

                 2.   Not possible to be specific about some symptoms, e.g. no way of coding leg pain - nearest is pain; i.e. not comprehensive - only a limited number of terms.

3.   Requires a lot of space on computer to accommodate full text.

Development of an in-house coding system or thesaurus

In the author's view the best advice to anyone wishing to construct such an in-house coding system or thesaurus is "don't", unless you have a lot of time and resources available. However, if such an exercise is considered essential, it is bound to take far longer than originally thought. It is vital that a number of the potential users of the system are involved in term selection and structuring, to develop a thesaurus that is acceptable to all users. The first step is to work out what types of concepts in the documents to be indexed are to be included, i.e. a faceted analysis. This will give an idea of how the terms themselves may be grouped together. The individual terms themselves should be collected either on cards or a computer file. They can be obtained from other thesauri, book indexes, any pre-existing card indexes and from staff working in the various areas. The preferred terms and their synonyms can all be included. The interrelationships between collected terms can then be analysed. It is recommended that medical advice is taken here so that terms can be slotted into the most appropriate place in the hierarchy; however, such advice is sometimes conflicting. Test indexing of a batch of documents is the next procedure, preferably by a number of system users. New terms can then be added in as necessary. The thesaurus must continue to develop as it is used and is thus never finished.

CODING SYSTEMS AND THESAURI FOR DRUGS

Introduction

Apart from the drug that is being evaluated in a clinical trial or the drug that is the subject of an adverse reaction report, patients are frequently receiving other medicines. In many cases other therapies are relevant to the clinical trial or could be alternative aetiological candidates for the ADR. Furthermore, there is always the possibility of drug-drug interactions. Other drugs must, therefore, be recorded on clinical trial record and ADR forms and the information processed.

There are a number of available coding systems for drugs which can assist in the handling of this data. None is perfect for the reasons discussed below and the user must decide what his needs are and which system best answers them. One of the problems in devising a system to classify and code drugs is that there are several fundamentally different ways of approaching the task. Classification can be based on chemical structures (e.g. benzodiazepines), pharmacological action (e.g. anxiolytics) or therapeutic use (e.g. minor tranquillisers). In some cases drugs which have the same pharmacological action, e.g. beta-adrenergic blockers may have many different indications, such as angina, hypertension, cardiac arrhythmias, prevention of myocardial reinfarction and migraine prophylaxis, but not all members of the class have the same indications. The user may wish to identify all patients receiving a beta-adrenergic blocker and this would not be possible if a therapeutic use classification only had been used. Alternatively, the user might wish to identify all patients receiving antihypertensives in which case several pharmacological groups would have to be used, although this does not necessarily mean that the patient was taking the drug for hypertension. This problem can be overcome by using two or more different classifications and having the facility to put a drug into several therapeutic categories. However, this probably means a complicated system, lengthy codes and more computer space for fairly limited rewards. In practice most users only really need a simple system as searches for other drugs are not generally a frequent requirement. In many cases users have devised their own simple codes rather than opt for a more complex available system. The previous comments on the development of an in-house coding system or thesaurus for adverse events and diseases also apply to drugs.

Available coding systems and thesauri for drugs

As with coding systems for adverse events and diseases there is no ideal system, and choice must meet user needs. This review is also not comprehensive and reflects the author's personal experience. The systems considered are:

> Aberdeen/Dundee Medicines Codes
> DHSS Drug Master Index
> MIMS
> WHO Drug Reference List
> Others - BNF, CSM and OXMIS drug codes

Aberdeen/Dundee Medicines Codes

The system was developed in 1972 by the Medicines Evaluation and Monitoring section of the Department of Community Medicine in the University of Aberdeen and the Pharmacy Department in the Aberdeen Royal Infirmary. The system now has over 6,000 entries and a growth rate of about 150 new codes per annum. The code consists of five digits, the first two indicating a therapeutic group and the last three identifying individual drugs. Drug names appear as both approved and proprietary, together with non-standard names and common mis-spellings, but all have the same five digit code. As each drug has a unique number, it can only be entered in one therapeutic area and drugs have been assigned to the area considered most important. This process has in some cases been fairly arbitrary and there are some inconsistencies, although there is now more continuity. An additional pharmacological classification consisting of a further two digits was later added, mainly at the request of the Dundee group. This is useful but has not solved all the problems and inconsistencies.

Advantages

1. Readily available system, including computer tape

2. Regular (monthly) updating

3. Very comprehensive for U.K. drugs

4. Therapeutic and pharmacological classification, although some deficiencies here (see Disadvantages)

5. Able to create new codes for users but there is some delay in this

6. Reasonably assured future

7. Manageable code length - 5 digits + 2 more if pharmacological grouping is desired

Disadvantages

1. Drugs are listed under only one therapeutic area. If a drug was being used for a secondary indication, this information will be lost as only the main therapeutic use is incorporated in the code, e.g. salbutamol when used in premature labour will still be coded 11008 where 11 = bronchodilators. This problem is partly overcome in some cases by use of the additional pharmacological grouping.

2. There are anomalies in the system due to past inconsistencies in creating codes.

3. Not so comprehensive for non U.K. drugs, but:

  (a) if it is a single drug substance that is also available in the U.K., the approved name could be used.

  (b) the number of overseas drugs in the system is increasing following requests from pharmaceutical companies.

  (c) new codes for overseas drugs could be created.

  (d) a general code for the group of drugs could be used if a specific code was not available, e.g. 60000 = Antacids.

4. Therapeutic and pharmacological classifications are not ideal.

Department of Health and Social Security (DHSS) Drug Master Index

The DHSS Drug Master Index is available in the U.K. from the DHSS Statistics and Research Division. It contains entries for drugs dispensed by contracting chemists and hospitals. Each drug is assigned a series of codes as follows:

A Drug number - this is up to 5 digits and has been allocated sequentially to each strength and form of a drug.

B Class of preparation - a single digit indicating whether the drug is generic or proprietary, etc.

C Therapeutic classification - 25 broad classifications, further sub-divided by another digit.

D Medicament classification - 2 digits indicating dosage form.

For each drug there is also a manufacturer's code (3 digits), a standard quantity unit and the year of introduction. The index presumably meets the needs of the DHSS but its other applications are limited for the reasons given below. It is planned that the Drug Master Index will be merged with the Prescription Pricing Authority system in about two years' time.

Advantages

1. Readily available system

2. Very comprehensive for U.K. drugs

3. Produced annually and updates available monthly

Disadvantages

1. Poor therapeutic classification. Drugs only listed under one indication - see also Aberdeen/Dundee Medicines Codes

2. Not intended for non U.K. drugs

3. Fairly complex code structure

MIMS (Monthly Index of Medical Specialities)

Although not intended as a system of drug codes, MIMS[284] does possess a pharmacological classification and therapeutic index. The pharmacological classification is simple and consists of numbers 1 to 18 (basically body systems) which is then further subdivided A to J. There is no unique code for each drug but every proprietary prescription product appears in the appropriate pharmacological group, or groups if there is more than one indication. MIMS may meet the needs of some users or may serve as a basis for development and modification of an in-house code.

Advantages

1. Simple and readily available

2. Published monthly - hence new products quickly incorporated

3.   Very good for U.K. proprietary prescription medicines

4.   Drugs appear in more than one pharmacological/therapeutic group, where appropriate

Disadvantages

1.   No unique code for each drug

2.   Not intended for non U.K. drugs, many OTC drugs and drugs in clinical trial

WHO - Drug Reference List

The Drug Reference List or Drug Dictionary[269] is a cross-index of drugs available from the W.H.O. Monitoring Programme of Adverse Reactions to Drugs and includes all drugs that have appeared on the ADR reports reviewed.   The drug appears as the preferred name, which is the international non-proprietary name (INN) in the case of single ingredient drugs and for multiple ingredient medicines the first reported name of the given combination.   Each drug is assigned a unique six digit number, a single letter classifying the type of drug name, e.g. INN, trade name, chemical name, etc., a two digit source code indicating the reference source where it was found and three letters which abbreviate the manufacturer's name.

There are both pharmacological and therapeutic classifications consisting of 21 and 24 main classes respectively and these are identified by a four character alphanumerical code.   There is provision for up to six pharmacological and six therapeutic classes for each drug.   There are now over 10,000 different drug names in the Drug Reference List.

Advantages

1.   Readily available system, including computer tape

2.   Comprehensive and international

3.   Good pharmacological and therapeutic classifications

4.   Able to list drugs in several pharmacological and therapeutic groups

Disadvantages

1.   May take a while for new drugs to be allocated codes and incorporated in the system

2.   Complex code structure, particularly if several pharmacological and therapeutic classifications are used

Others

BNF (British National Formulary)

The BNF[285] classifies drugs and preparations in a similar way to MIMS, i.e. basically under fifteen body systems which are then further subdivided. This could also be used as a coding system for groups of drugs or an in-house system and unique drug codes could be developed from it. The advantages and disadvantages are much the same as with MIMS.

CSM (Committee on Safety of Medicines)

The CSM use a 6-digit code to facilitate the evaluation of adverse reaction reports[286]. The first two digits broadly classify the drug into one of approximately 50 groups primarily according to similarity of therapeutic action. The latter 4 digits classify the drug further according to chemical structure. Each drug also has a unique identity number which is up to 4 digits and is allocated sequentially.

OXMIS drug codes

These codes have never been published but are used by the Oxford Community Health Project[287]. They consist of a prefix, e.g. A - approved name, P - proprietary name, C - compound, followed by a four-digit code. There is no classification within this code which severely limits its applications.

OUTPUT AND ANALYSIS OF ADR DATA

Basically, the users must decide their own output requirements, hence it is only possible to suggest a few ideas and point out some pitfalls. The chosen system should be designed after required outputs and analyses have been specified or be sufficiently flexible to cope with many output formats. Many software systems are capable of straightforward numerical outputs but more sophisticated systems can produce histograms, graphical representations, and carry out further numerical and statistical analyses on the data. As always, computer output must be interpreted with care.

An example of useful output from a controlled clinical trial is the hypothical adverse event profile shown in Figure A. The number of patients experiencing certain common, symptomatic, events on both active drug and placebo are represented for comparative purposes. In this example, the difference in incidence of two events is statistically significant, rash at P=0.05 and diarrhoea at P less than 0.01. This does not mean that all recorded cases of rash or diarrhoea were due to the study drug, as there was a background incidence of these events in the patients on placebo but it suggests that some of the events are drug related and that these cases deserve further individual attention. Conversely, it does not mean that all cases of headache, dizziness, anxiety, vomiting, fatigue, nausea or constipation are unrelated to the study drug.

Figure A: Adverse event profile - drug v placebo

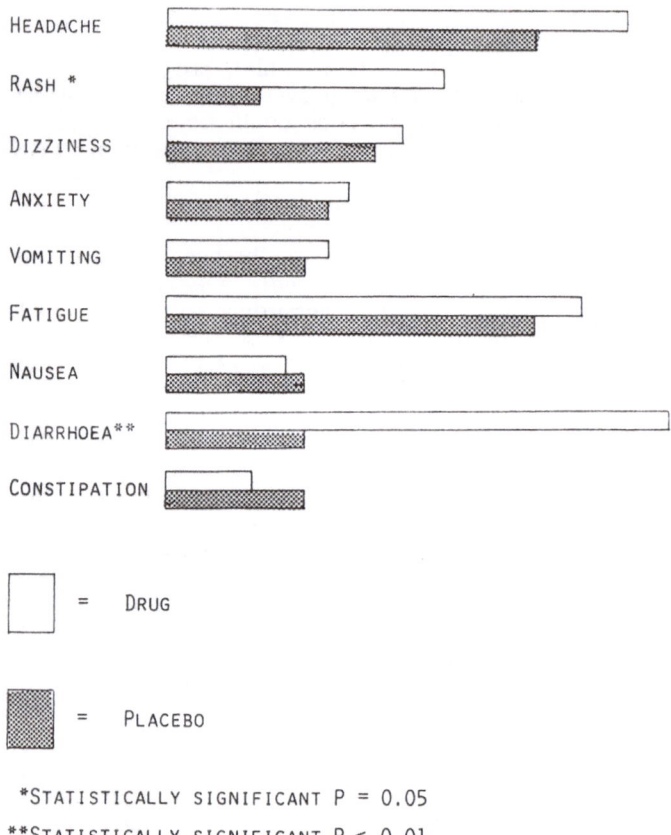

Another hypothetical example of data ouput is shown in figure B where the occurrence of a particular ADR is analysed with respect to the age of the patients. This sort of analysis should be undertaken as older patients are often at greater risk of developing ADRs. In the example given, elderly patients, particularly those in their seventh decade, appear to be most likely to experience the ADR. However, this histogram should be compared alongside the histogram of the ages of patients receiving the drug to see whether the patterns are different. This should be simple for clinical trial reports but often presents difficulties in interpreting spontaneous reports as denominator data is notoriously poor. Hazards with interpreting such data are illustrated by the apparent fall in the number of cases in patients in their ninth decade. This does not mean that great age confers protection, but rather, that fewer patients in this age group were treated!

Figure B: Occurrence of an ADR by age

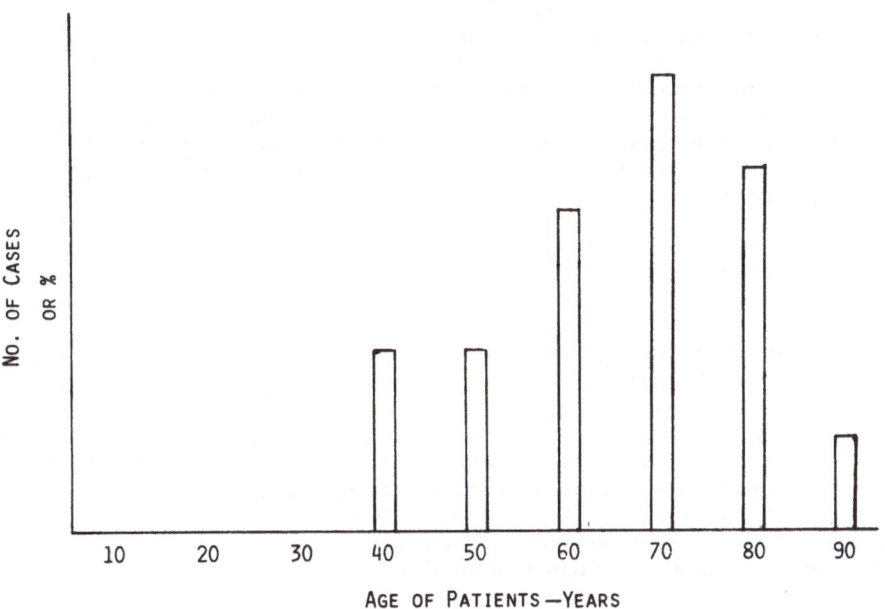

Figure C: Occurrence of an ADR by time to onset

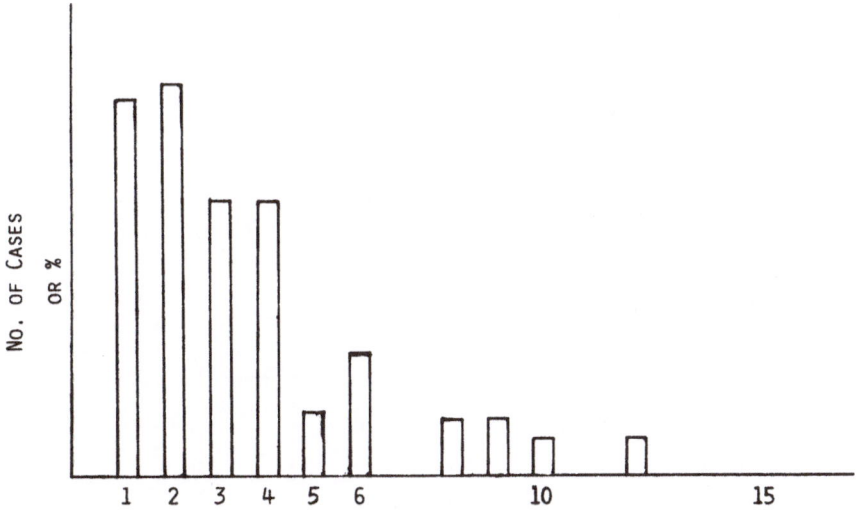

Figure C shows a further example of data output illustrating the occurrence of an ADR by its time to onset in days. The time taken from a patient starting a drug to experiencing a particular ADR is often fairly consistent, a narrow range in time to onset could suggest a causal relationship. In this example the time to onset in the majority of cases was in the first four days of treatment. This could suggest causality with the short time to onset probably meaning that the ADR is a type A reaction i.e. an exaggerated pharmacological response. However, it could also be the result of the patient's or doctor's initial enthusiasm on starting a clinical trial.

CONCLUSIONS

This chapter has outlined the sources of ADR data, their differences and some of their limitations. As emphasised throughout, the choice of computer hardware and software depends on many factors and only general guidance can be given. Similarly the characteristics, advantages and disadvantages of some coding systems and thesauri have been described but selection depends on user needs and preference. It is vital for the various users to define exact needs and agree on these; however, it is recommended that a degree of flexibility is built into a system as requirements frequently change with time.

ACKNOWLEDGEMENTS

I wish to thank my colleagues who provided constructive comment and advice on various aspects of this chapter. The Wellcome Research Laboratories ADR transcription document is reproduced in the appendix by kind permission from Mr David E. Smith.

9
The Ethical Problems of a Pharmaceutical Physician

Many major pharmaceutical companies of many nations, including the U.K., have been criticised for unethical behaviour in relation to ADR[288,289,290]. The pharmaceutical industry has been criticised by Shapiro[291] in the following terms: "I suggest, and in fact insist, that anyone engaged in the academic study of adverse reactions has to treat companies as potential adversaries, to maintain a distance from them and be required that any research must be independent of them"; and by Temple[292] (Bureau of the F.D.A.), "Bias exists everywhere but the difference is that the bias of the drug industry is always in one direction"; by Fülgraff[293] (President of the Bundesgesundheitsamtes): "Our experience is that many manufacturers are at least dangerous or ambiguous partners and they will continue to be so as long as they incline to the policy of appeasement against adverse reactions and to a purely defensive attitude in the reactions towards newly suspected ADRs". In the 1983 meeting of the American Drug Information Association, Robert Temple, the acting Director of New Drug Evaluation, said whilst talking on the new regulation guidelines for New Drug Applications and referring to the form used for these applications (356H): "The form 356H also requires something called an evaluation of safety and effectiveness. That evaluation has to do some of the following things: it has to summarise separately the favourable and unfavourable evidence for each claim in labelling. I was thinking to myself as I read that that I do not think that I have ever seen a summary of the unfavourable evidence, at least not so identified - even though that is right in the regulations as a requirement. Anyway, it is supposed to reference the location of detailed data for each of the favourable and unfavourable data. The evaluation is supposed to tabulate all side effects or adverse experiences by age, sex and dosage formulation, whether they are considered drug-related, and the tabulation is also supposed to show whether administration of the drug was stopped. It is supposed to give the investigator's name and the location of the report. The overall requirements are not very detailed about how to make an NDA but the part referring to the tabulation of side effects is fairly detailed and again, as I was going over that, I noted that it is not uncommon for that aspect of the regulation not to be fulfilled in a submission.   The tabulation plainly calls for reports of adverse experiences - it does not say anything about adverse drug effects." This suggests that some bias still exists.

The bias may be conscious or unconscious and be shown either in:

1.   interpretation of the regulations

2.   the presentation of facts

3.   opinion and/or comment on the facts

and one needs to ask certain questions if one is to detect bias.

1.   **Interpretation of the regulations**

If one contrasts the exact and defined terminology used by the F.D.A. (see page 14)) with the U.K. regulations (see page 134, 135, paragraph 3) "..... inform the licensing authority of any information received by him that casts doubt" (U.K.) and paragraph 4 "the licence holder shall maintain a record of reports of which he is aware, of adverse effects" (U.K.). "Casting doubt" is a matter of opinion and it could be argued that an "adverse effect" implies a certain causality between drug and event. There is much more room for bias in the interpretation of the U.K. regulations than in the F.D.A. regulations. Both F.D.A. regulations and U.K. regulations allow for "inspection by a person authorised by the licensing authority" (U.K.), whereas Chapter 1: F.D.A. para 310.300, subpart D "Records and reports", paragraph 65d from the draft guidelines for use of FDA 1639 states "the applicant shall permit such officers to have access to and copy and verify any records and reports....." with a threat of withdrawal of a drug's approval for any transgressors.

Although both authorities have the right to inspect the records of the licence holders and, therefore, to check whether any bias has taken place in the interpretation of the regulations, there is a difference in the practice of the authorities. The F.D.A. regularly inspects the records of the pharmaceutical company and does not hesitate to do so outside the U.S.A., i.e. in the U.K. but I do not believe that the "record of reports" of a single product licence holder in the U.K. has ever been inspected by a person authorised by the U.K. licensing authority.   The results of the F.D.A. inspections are available under the Freedom of Information Act and make interesting reading.

2.   **Presentation of the facts**

Reports on ADR to the various regulatory authorities need to be presented in an easy-to-read structured form. It is not feasible or sensible to include a photocopy of every piece of evidence, since in some cases there are box-loads of data. Bias may be shown in the selection of the facts to be presented or in the way in which the data has been processed. The use of vague adjectives or phrases, such as "a few cases", "a small number of reports", "isolated cases", "some reports", in place of exact numbers should arouse suspicion. The authenticity of the facts can be undermined by criticism of the manner in which they were obtained. Justifiable criticism should be given of those facts which are against drug involvement as well as those which support a drug involvement. Since information concerning a single case may be collected over many months, it is difficult to decide when to close a case and when to report it to the various authorities. Some reports may be delayed until a suitable time, i.e. after a particular submission of data for marketing.

3. Opinion and comment

Since the value of an opinion will vary according to the status and experience of the person giving the opinion, every opinion should be followed by their name and status so that they can be questioned as to the basis of the opinion, i.e. has he/she read all the data or merely a summary. Comment or opinion by non-medically qualified staff or medically qualified staff with little clinical experience should be avoided. The use of a "devil's advocate" to read all reports before submission to an outside authority might reduce bias if the devil's advocate has sufficient authority and integrity.

Some drugs which have been found to have serious ADR have been withdrawn from the market but there are a few which, although withdrawn from some markets, remain on other markets. A justification for this could be that the characteristics of the two populations differ. The physician responsible for the ADR of his company's products must satisfy himself that such a justification exists and that positive evidence has been published. Where a drug has been removed from sophisticated markets where monitoring of ADR is reasonable, and left on the market in under-developed countries or those where ADR monitoring is non-existent, there is unlikely to be any ethical justification. Consumer interpol can supply a list of products which remain on selected markets[294].

In the light of these criticisms it is of the greatest importance that the pharmaceutical physician has high integrity in order to resist those actions which are not motivated by concern for the patient. The responsibility of an ADR physician is to the patient(s) above all else. All actions must be tested by the touchstone "Is this in the interest of the patient(s)?". The ADR physician cannot separate himself from the dangers produced by unethical marketing, and part of his duty should be to inspect all data sheets for his company's products for all countries where they are marketed, to ensure that they are consistent with known properties of the drug and that local changes in wording are justified.

It has been suggested[295] that, when a doctor within the industry is the victim of what he considers "unfair dismissal" because of a stand he has taken on a particular issue for ethical reasons, the machinery should be in existence for representation to be made on his behalf to the company management. A joint team from the British Medical Association and the Association for Medical Advisers in the Pharmaceutical Industry can now tackle this problem on behalf of their members. However, a pharmaceutical company is unlikely to make any clear connection between the physician's response to an ethical problem and his dismissal. The pressures on a physician to keep silent are likely to be subtle and will rarely be presented in ethical terms.

10
Update

This chapter has been added at the last minute to ensure that the book is up-to-date and, therefore, all new references are included in the text.

Chapter 1

Introduction

Placebo (page 21)

The leader in The Lancet (No. 8365/624, of 31st December 1983) entitled "Shall I please" quotes that there is no evidence for an opioid component in placebo analgesia and goes on to say that there is no reason to believe that the placebo effect has a single specific mechanism.

McDonald, C.J. and Mazzuca, S.A. in an article entitled "How much of the placebo effect is really statistical regression" (Statistics in Medicine, 1983, 2, 417-427) argue that most improvements attributed to the placebo effect are actually instances of statistical regression, i.e. a tendency of extreme measures to move closer to the mean when they are repeated. This obviously cannot account for the adverse effects of placebo where what was normal becomes abnormal.

Chapter 2

The methodology of the collection of adverse events

The quality of life (page 38)

Chronic disease requiring chronic therapy necessitates the addition of time as a factor in the cost/benefit ratio. For each day the quality of life can be scored and added together giving a total score or aggregated Health Status Index (HSI). The score can be obtained by asking the patient what reduced life expectation he/she would trade for restoration of health. C. J. Bulpitt has dealt with the quality of life in hypertensive patients in a chapter in "Hypertensive Cardiovascular Disease. Pathophysiology and treatment" (edited by Amery, A. and published by Martinus Nijhoff in 1982). The same author deals with the subject in a wider context in his own book (see bibliography).

"Measuring and analysing quality of life in cancer clinical trials: a review" by Fayers, P.M. and Jones, D.R. (Statistics in Medicine, 1983, 2, 429-446) is an excellent review which has extensive references covering quality of life measurements in fields other than that of cancer.

Clinicians' evaluation of laboratory results

An alternative to the system (e) [page 35] where the two categories refer to the normal range is to have two categories related to their clinical significance; either there has been a change of clinical significance or any change is not clinically significant. This would entail a single box for each value, i.e. SGOT before, during and at the end of the study, and it would only require a tick if any change is of clinical significance. If any individual value(s) is ticked then an overall comment should be given on the complete laboratory data for that patient.

Visual analogue scale as an alternative to a checklist

The advantage of a visual analogue scale is that the patient does not attach a verbal label to his judgements. A study of antihistamines compared a checklist containing 24 items with the Somesthetic Inventory (an analogue scale for 54 body feelings). The former showed no significant differences for the 24 items whilst the latter showed significant effects, i.e. sedation by one of the antihistamines which was supported by objective data (Lundberg, P.K., Assessment of drugs' side effects. Visual analogue scale versus checklist format. Perceptual and Motor Skills, 1980, 50, 1067-1073).

Chapter 3

Assessment of adverse events (page 55)

In the latter half of 1983 there were three international and one French meeting which dealt with this subject.

1.   Droit et Pharmacie meeting, Paris, 26th and 27th September:

Dr. Cornelli presented his scoring system for the assessment of adverse events. He is the medical director of the Italian pharmaceutical company Recordati SpA, Milano, Via Civitali 1, Italy.

Dr. Cornelli considers five factors:

1.   Dosage - can the disease be treated with the drug and is the dosage correct.

2.   Pathology - the frequency of the adverse event if it is a symptom or syndrome occurring in patients suffering from the disease under treatment with the drug.

3.   Concomitant therapy - present or absent, with a safe or non-safe drug and whether it can cause the adverse event.

4.   Chronology - whether the event occurred during therapy, after or is relatively correlated.

5.   Rechallenge - positive, doubtful, impossible or negative.

Each of these five factors is scored 1 to 4 and different total scores are equated to the different final assessments - definite, almost definite, probable, possible, very doubtful or unrelated. The method was published in the chapter "Example of Naproxen". A multicentre Italian trial in the Vol II of 'Essais cliniques postmarketing. Les études de phase IV' published by Droit et Pharmacie.

2.   The American Drug Information Association Adverse Reaction Workshop took place in Arlington, Virginia from .30th October to 2nd November. This will probably be published as Volume 13 of the 1984 Drug Information Association Journal.

      (a)   Dr. W. Castle of I.C.I. (U.K.) presented her pictorial/numerical method for different adverse event patterns.

      (b)   Dr. A. Ruskin circulated his algorithms:

             (i)   A drug-event algorithm (appendix page 234) and
             (ii)   The drug death algorithm (page 235)

      (c)   Dr. A. Emanueli gave details of his revised method (page 236

3.   The third meeting was a small workshop organised by the Active Permanent Workshop of Imputologists (A.P.W.I.) held in Paris between the 28th and 30th November. Many of the authors of individual algorithms spoke on their own methods and various improvements, most of which had been presented at previous meetings. Although the discussions did not lead to an algorithm which would meet with everybody's approval, the need to devise such an algorithm was considered necessary. A small nucleus of members, headed by Professor Lane, has proposed a three-year programme to devise and test such a method.

The fourth meeting was the "Cinquièmes Journées Françaises de Pharma covigilance" which was organised by the Association des Centres d Pharmacogivilance Hospitalière on the 24th and 25th November 198 Madame C. Bastin gave a paper entitled "Imputabilité automatique de effets indésirables des médicaments a l'aide d'une méthode informatisé d'analyse de correspondence (Bastín, Ch., Wertheimer, P., Smith, P.R. and Venulet, J., Adverse drug reactions - a computer assisted application of correspondence analysis for automatic causality assessment).   Using Dr. Venulet's method (page 46) as a basis, the Ciba-Geigy experts evaluated 204 separate cases and then, with the aid of a computer, the various factors were assessed by correspondence analysis and the strength of evidence calculated and this was used subsequently for the discriminant analysis of a separate set of 100 cases. In 60% of the cases this evaluative assessment of causality was identical with that obtained through the analysis. I did not understand the statistics of the method but an English version of the paper was given at the A.P.W.I. meeting and this reinforced my feelings of ignorance. The paper will be published next year and I will ask a kind statistician to guide me through it.

The latter part of 1983 saw five papers published on comparison of different methods of assessment.

The first two by Lagier et al (Lagier, G., Vincens, M., Lefebure, B. & Frelon, J.M., Assessment of individual ADR.   Comparison of Methods, Therapie, 1983, 38, 295-302).   The first contains his method (methode appréciative ponderée) and the second compares the logic of ten methods with that of his own method developed at the Hopital Fernand Widal Centre de Pharmacovigilance.

The Bordeaux Centre de Pharmacovigilance has proposed a theoretical model for the assessment of ADR and analyses the different methods used for comparison.   The Kappa test is favoured by them for the comparison of two methods (Père, J.C., Begaud, B., Haramburu, F. & Albin, H., Methode d'étude des effets indésirables des médicaments, Thérapie (In Press)).   There is a second part to the paper, Comparison de cinq méthodes d'imputabilité au moyen d'observations simulées par informatique.   Resumes et communications, vème journées Françaises de pharmacovigilance, Nov. 1983, 2-27, which compares five different methods with 1,134 adverse events simulated by computer, the concordance always being better between two algorithms than between any algorithm and chance.   For the Kappa and weighted Kappa test the concordance was never more than "moderate".

The other two papers do not compare the algorithms by their results on a selection of cases but discuss the areas of disagreement and difference. Hasford reviews six papers which have measured the level of disagreement concerning the assessment of an adverse event without using an algorithm which ranges from 37% to 80%.   He goes on to discuss the different algorithms, their advantages and disadvantages, and certain types of adverse event which are not amenable to solving by the present methods. (Hasford, J., Causality assessment of suspected adverse drug reactions. Decision algorithms, applicability and statistical aspects.   World conference on Clinical Pharmacology and Therapeutics, Washington DC, 1983).

Hutchinson, Kramer and colleagues from Montreal used their algorithm as a means of discovering areas of disagreement.   (Hutchinson, T.A., Flegel, K.M. et al, Reasons for disagreement in the standardised assessment of suspected adverse drug reactions, Clin. Pharmac. & Ther., 1983, 34 (4), 421–426). Two of them used the algorithm on 80 adverse events and recorded 66% agreement. Not surprisingly, they found that disagreement on judgmental questions about three times as numerous as those on factual questions. The five questions with the highest rate of disagreement were:

1.   Bibliography of drug/event - 23%.

2.   Pre-existing condition commonly followed by the event - 23%

3.   Does the event commonly occur in this type of patient without recognisable cause - 38%

4.   Was the timing inconsistent with an ADR to this drug - 24%

5.   Was the timing as expected for an ADR to this drug - 36%.

I have paraphrased the questions and given the percentage disagreement. The authors also listed the areas where there is disagreement due to poor sources of information:

1.   Lists of adverse events that are well-known to occur with various drugs.

2.   Symptoms that can be expected with various diseases and without diseases.

3.   The expected timing for a variety of adverse drug reactions.

Chapter 4

Phase 1 Studies

The irreproachable record for the study of new drugs in volunteers referred to on page 66 was marred in 1984. The Times of Monday June 11th page 3 reported that a student volunteer who had taken part in a trial of a tranquillizing drug subsequently developed aplastic anaemia and later died and that an Irish student volunteer died 15 minutes after an injection of a new drug. Scrip No 904 (June 11th) page 7 stated that the drug involved was an anti-arrhythmic drug EXPOXINDINE. The Times of June 12th reported that the Royal College of Physicians had set up a group of experts which would review guidelines on the testing of medical drugs on volunteers.

Chapter 5

Postmarketing Surveillance

Having described the situation regarding PMS up to the present, we must look at current thought as to future policies.

1. There are regulations in five countries requiring reports on the safety of products after marketing at set intervals, namely the U.S.A., West Germany, Japan, Italy and Taiwan. This will tend to spread to other countries and will have an ever-increasing importance within pharmaceutical companies requiring a considerable increase in personnel.

2. The spate of drug withdrawals between 1980 and 1984 - ticrynafen, benoxaprofen, zomepirac, zelmedine, Osmosin, flosint and oxphenbutazone - has stirred regulatory authorities to close any loopholes and examine PMS anew. It is necessary to look at each country separately.

United Kingdom

A working party has been set up by the Committee on Safety of Medicines (C.S.M.) to look at adverse reactions, its terms of reference being "to consider how best the C.S.M. should fulfil its statutory function of promoting the collection and investigation of information relating to adverse reactions for the purpose of enabling it to give advice on safety, quality or efficacy of medicinal products and to make recommendations".

The work has been split into two stages; the first "to review the present system relating to ADR and to consider how this can be improved", and the second will consider, in the longer term, additional ideas about drug monitoring, for example event monitoring and record linkage, as well as the full potentialities of new information technology.

The report on Stage 1 made the following recommendations:

1. Improvement of the present yellow card system, including advising doctors about what they should report (see **page 137**).

2. The rejection of making reporting mandatory.

3. Exploring the possibility of setting up organ-specific registers similar to the A.M.A. blood dyscrasia registry.

4. The possibility of pharmacists reporting ADR should be considered but the direct reporting by patients was not advisable.

5. That further regional centres should not be organised until there is evidence that the reporting rate in the regions of the present centres has increased as a result of these centres.

6.   That formal monitoring after a period of five years, or after prescriptions for 5,000,000 patients have been given, is unlikely to detect any significant hazards and, therefore, the possibility of limited monitoring should be considered.

7.   That guidelines should be circulated to the pharmaceutical industry clarifying the extent of the industry's legal obligation to report and the C.S.M.'s wishes. This would also include guidance on ADR in drugs under clinical trial and the reporting of non-U.K. data.

8.   Consideration should be given as to how the Committee could have easy access to information about ADR occurring in other countries.

9.   There should be discussions with the A.B.P.I. as to how the industry could promote doctors' awareness of ADR, including training sales representatives to give more information about ADR to doctors and adding a remark about reporting ADR to advertisements for drugs containing new chemical entities.

The report contains a total of 29 recommendations. No doubt the revised MAL 2 and 4 which are due in 1984 will give substance to some of these recommendations. The second stage report is expected during 1984.

A workshop was held in October 1983 in London entitled "Monitoring for Adverse Drug Reactions" under the auspices of the U.K. Centre for Medicines Research. The possibility of setting up morbidity registers for specific disease areas by specialist societies was discussed. Once a hypothesis has been generated by spontaneous reporting or cohort studies, it was thought that a record linkage system held most promise as a subsequent hypothesis testing scheme. However, the costs would be high unless the system also served some other function. (The results of the workshop will be published under the same title during 1984 by MTP Press and edited by Professor S. Walker and Professor Sir A. Goldberg.)

Post-marketing Surveillance

The British Medical Journal of the 24th March 1984 p.911-914 contained an article entitled "Post-marketing surveillance: Practical experience with Ketotifen" by Maclay, W. P., Crowder, D., Spiro, S. and Turner, P. with a useful discussion of the problems involved.

Correspondence in the British Medical Journal of the 24th May p.879 by Professor M. D. Rawlins and in the issue of the 14th April p.1155-6 by Dr W. H. W. Inman and Dr E. S. Snell reviewed post-marketing studies and the problems involved in the yellow card and green card systems (P.E.M.) and the industry's point of view of the yellow card system.

The Lancet of May 19th 1984 p.1116 contained an article by Professor P. Turner entitled "Food and drugs: Why different approaches to their safety?" which suggested a form of conditional approval for new drugs similar to that used with food additives. Restriction of marketing activity was advocated during the long-term safety studies, i.e. such as that undertaken at the Southampton drug surveillance unit (P.E.M.).

The editor of Scrip, Dr P. Brown, writing in the Scrip No 902 of June 4th 1984 p.2 gave 6 reasons for the growing disenchantment of the pharmaceutical companies with PMS studies and went on to suggest that a small group of experts appointed by health authorities could be given the ongoing responsibility for giving an authorative view on any question relating to the product's safety profile.   These experts would be specialists in the therapeutic area to which the drug related and they would oversee the collection and evaluation of evidence of the drug's safety for at least the first 3 years after marketing.

The A.B.P.I. distributed copies of their guidelines (Ref 435/84) which had been formulated to assist member companies on the ethical aspects of conducting company sponsored PMS schemes.   Reference was made to these in the British Medical Journal of 14th April 1984, 288, 1156.

Guidelines

1.   Any prospective PMS study, sponsored by a pharmaceutical company, which includes the writing of a prescription by a medical practitioner for that company's products, must not include the offer of any financial or other inducement for the writing of that prescription or the subsequent completion of a patient record form or other similar documentation.   In addition such studies must not represent a form of sales promotion.

2.   In retrospective PMS studies, payment for completing patient record forms or other similar documentation may be acceptable provided that the study does not represent a form of sales promotion.

3.   A company may be requested by the Licensing Authority to undertake some form of prospective PMS. In this instance provided the protocol has been discussed with and formally approved by the Licensing Authority and is not a form of sales promotion, the offer of a reasonable fee to the medical practitioner to complete a patient record form or similar documentation may be acceptable if conditions of payment have been discussed with the Licensing Authority.

Royal College of General Practice PMS

Professor J.G.R. Howie, referring to the Medical Surveillance Organisation (M.S.O.) multicentre clinical appraisal study (page 107),   wrote in the Journal of the Royal College of General Practice (vol. 33, No. 257, December 1983) "Any attempt to comment in a clinically useful way about efficacy and acceptability on the basis of a study which does not use a standard alternative preparation and is not double-blind must be suspect". He went on to comment on one of the Royal College of General Practice M.S.O. studies that "surveillance can only be effective if it is substantially more active than that being progressed in this study".

United States

Dr. Anello of the F.D.A., when speaking on Phase 4 studies in Paris in September 1983 (The use, design and limitations of selected Phase 4 studies in the U.S.A., Droit et Pharmacie, vol. III), reviewed 54 NDAs for which marketing approval had been made conditional on initiation of post-marketing studies:

1. Better quantifying the ADR in the population at risk (19 NDAs)

2. Testing in children (13 NDAs)

3. Long-term use (5 NDAs)

4. Comparison with other drugs (5 NDAs)

5. Other indications (2 NDAs)

6. Abuse potential (2 NDAs)

7. Bioavailability (2 NDAs)

8. Effects on specific end organs (2 NDAs)

9. Teratology (2 NDAs)

10. Better establish the dose (2 NDAs)

Although the analysis of the three American company-initiated PMS schemes reached the conclusion that this type of study should not be repeated, this does not imply that PMS cohort schemes should be abandoned. Dr. Anello suggests that, where there is a specific problem and the drug is of limited use in certain populations, then a cohort study or cohort design may be the best type of PMS. However, it should:

(a) have an appropriate comparison group

(b) be large enough to detect pre-specified risks

(c) assume complete or near complete follow-up

(d) identify pre-specified adverse reactions or events

(e) be analysed using a method that takes into account the potential for losses to follow-up and time dependent risks (Life Table Analysis).

Contained within the paper by Anello was Appendix 1 - a paper by Robert T. O'Neill entitled "Assessing adverse event rates in clinical trials as a function of duration of treatment exposure" which developed Life Table Analysis.

America

The PMS using Medicaid (see page 109) is known as COMPASS (Computerised Airline Medicaid Pharmaceutical Analysis and Surveillance System) and has been developed by Health Information Designs Inc. with funding from the F.D.A. The first study relates gastro-intestinal toxicity of 7 non-steroidal anti-inflammatory drugs using 88,644 patients.

A letter in JAMA of February 10th 1984 Vol. 251 No 6 p.729-730 from the Upjohn Company discussed the paper by Rossi et al.[250] on the comparison of phase IV studies with spontaneous reporting methods. The reply from Rossi et al. stated that a comparison of incidence rates of common adverse effects in clinical trials with these in a phase IV study showed an almost 18-fold difference (15.8% in clinical trials and 0.9% in phase IV studies). This correspondence highlights the problems of PMS undertaken by American pharmaceutical companies.

The Upjohn Company's medication monitoring programme uses a computer-assisted telephone interviewing system for direct patient contact in postmarketing drug surveillance (Crawley, J.A., Hochard, R.A. and Krieger, K.S., The role of computer assisted telephone interviewing in clinical research, Clin. Res. Practices and Drug. Reg. Affairs, 1983, 1 (4), 303-311).

France

The arrival of the previous Head of the Bordeaux Pharmacovigilance Centre, Professor Dangoumau, as the Pharmacy and Medicines Director, will have far-reaching effects on the postmarketing surveillance in France. This is likely to involve a strengthening of the regional centres with a stronger central organisation. Clinical pharmacologists - an almost unknown species in France - will be built into a specialty. PMS, he believes, should be essentially an industrial affair. He also wishes to build up a capability to undertake various epidemiological studies in France. Professor Dangoumau has said that PMS in France now needs to be restructured and reinforced if it is to cope with a considerable amount of work in the next few years. This suggests that important changes are imminent in France and it is likely that reporting of ADR will become obligatory and that reporting sources will include pharmacists and nurses, the ADR on established drugs going to the regional centres, whilst those on new drugs to the National Pharmacovigilance Centre via the pharmaceutical company. The pharmaceutical manufacturers' association (S.N.I.P.) has established a code of practice on pharmacovigilance which is binding on its members (Circular No. 9974, Pharmacovigilance 03 Syndicat Nationale de l'Industrie Pharmaceutique, 88 rue de la Faisanderie 75782 Paris 16).

Germany

Scrip reports in the May 23 1984 issue No. 899 p.7 that the West German industry association (B.P.I.) proposed that:-

(1)   All member companies be obliged to report immediately all adverse drug reactions which are potentially lethal or likely to cause permanent injury, to the B.G.A. and the Medicines commission of the medical profession. This concerns all products regardless of whether the adverse drug reaction was already known or being reported for the first time.

(2)   Each company to appoint a specially qualified representative for adverse drug reactions, their names to be known to the B.G.A., Medicines Commission and the B.P.I. secretariat.

Nordic Countries

Merkantil-Tryckeriet AB of Uppsala published in 1984 'suspected ADRs reported in the Nordic Countries 1981' which contains the numbers of each reaction, using preferred terms, and the number of cases in each of the five Nordic Countries.

Italy

Postmarketing Regulations

The law has been amended (28th July 1984) and the amendments come into force on January 1st 1985.

The annual postmarketing reports required after the first two years have to be supplied indefinitely rather than for only three years as hitherto.

The notification of fatal adverse reactions must be 'timely', which means as soon as the company is in possession of 'adequate information elements' and any way not later than 15 days after the time that the company knows the outcome of the reaction.

A new adverse drug reaction form is introduced and the notes accompanying it say that even minor effects must be reported – and these are those which constitute in any manner a sign of non-tolerance of the drug even if they have been described in the literature or in the illustrative leaflet.

The periodic reports must have an appendix containing a copy of the new form for each case and similarly a copy of the WHO form contained in 'International Adverse Drug Reaction Monitoring. Guide to participating countries'.

Testing many hypotheses - the statistical problem

Earlier in the book (page 13 and page 106) the problem of statistical analysis of numerous variables when comparing two groups was raised. The only suggested approach at that time was to reduce the level of significance of each subgroup so that the sum of the separate subgroups remained as before and this was done by dividing the P value by the number of classes (subgroups) examined with a resultant loss of sensitivity. This is the Bonferroni adjustment. A recent review paper in the Annals of Internal Medicine, published in January 1984 (vol. 100, pages 122 to 129 by Cupples, L.A., Heeken, T., Schatzkin, A, & Colton, T.) entitled "Multiple testing of hypotheses in comparing two groups" discusses the problem and puts forward three methods for tackling it:

(a)   Hotellings T^2

(b)   Discriminant analysis

(c)   Logistic regression

The authors discussed their various uses as a preliminary step with the subsequent use of Bonferroni's adjustment. The use of Bonferroni's adjustment when there are many variables, however, still leaves unsolved problems and the authors in their discussion say "researchers should be wary of comparing groups on many variables". Finally, the paper also mentions the problems of the multiple laboratory tests and the meaning of the occasional abnormal. Although these advances in the statistical management of monitoring many variables are very helpful, the final stage remains a clinical problem.

Chapter 7

Regulations

In January 1984 the Department of Health and Social Security (D.H.S.S.), U.K. wrote to each product licence holder via a Medicines Act Information Letter" [Mail 39], clarifying the present legal requirements:

> Companies are required to report all adverse effects associated with recently introduced products within the U.K. to their products within one month; a similar requirement to report all serious effects exists in respect of other products. When a serious effect occurs abroad, the company is required to report it without delay".

Drug Regulations

CMR NEWS is issued by the Centre for Medicines Research (an organisation established by the A.B.P.I. in 1981 as an independent scientific research unit to undertake research into the development and the safe use of medicines). In Vol.2 No.1 Spring 1984 it gives details of a WHO workshop on the effects of drug regulations. A book entitled "The Effects of Drug Regulations" edited by Drs G. Dukes and A. Smith will be published later that year and reflects the contents of the workshop. Professor S. Walker directs CMR from Woodmansterne Rd, Carshalton, Surrey SM5 4DS. A leader in the Lancet of March 31st 1984 page 718 entitled "When drug regulation fails" refers to the same WHO workshop and reviews its discussions and refers to some of the drugs withdrawn in the past year.

UK Regulations October 1984

Since Dr R. Penn checked the section on the UK regulations, MAIL 41 (Medicines Act Information Letter) has been published revoking the previous standard and special directions. The new directions are given in considerable detail.

The letter also states that reports of suspected reactions should contain:

1.   The name (or an identifying code) of the patient.

2.   The reporting doctor's name and address.

3.   The names of the drugs taken by the patient.

4.   The details of the reaction.

Suspected reactions should be confirmed in writing to the company by the doctor or dentist and, where the report is only verbal the company should ask for it to be substantiated in writing before reporting it. The company must not, however, wait for the outcome of the reaction before reporting it and should not draw distinctions between 'conceivable' and 'suspect' reactions to justify failing to report some reactions. Reports of cases of reactions published in the standard scientific literature need not be reported by the company.

Premarketing Adverse Reaction Reports

A.   Originating from the UK

1.   Products subject to clinical trial certificates (CTC).

'Any information which casts doubt on the continued validity of the data submitted with the application for the CTC in relation to the safety of the product in its proposed indication' must be reported to the licensing authority. Serious reactions should be submitted immediately whilst other reports should be provided in summary form at the end of the trial. All investigators must be informed of serious unpredictable reactions. If a study is discontinued the licensing authority must be notified and the reasons given.

'Serious' is defined as fatal, life-threatening, disabling or incapacitating' (the examples given on page 137 remain the same but with the exclusion of unexplained lack of effect or paradoxical effect).

2.   Products subject to clinical trial exemption (CTX).

All reactions must be reported forthwith. Speed in reporting is particularly important with serious reactions. All investigators should be informed of serious unpredicable reactions occurring in the trials.

B.   Originating from outside the UK

1.   Products subject to a CTC.

All serious and unpredictable reactions should be reported immediately. Other reactions should be reported in summary form either at the end of the UK trials or in any product licence application.

2.   Products subject to a CTX.

All reactions must be reported forthwith. Speed in reporting is particularly important with serious reactions.

Product Licence Applications (PLA)

Summaries of all adverse reactions reported to the company from clinical trials anywhere in the world must be submitted. This also applies to the period between submitting the PLA and hearing the result of the application. This applies to patients in clinical trials and also to individual patients treated on the clinicians' own responsibility outside the trial protocol. All clinical events reported to the company as adverse reactions by the responsible clinician whether or not they believe them to be caused by the product and whether or not they are specified in the trial protocol must be reported to the licensing authority.

In addition summaries of serious and unpredictable reactions occurring in other countries where the product is already licensed, including anecdotal reports and those from any postmarketing studies, must be submitted with the application.

Postmarketing Adverse Reaction Reports

A.   Originating from the UK

1.   New products.

These should be marked in the data sheet with a solid inverted triangle ▼. Special reporting is required on these products for four years after licensing. The licensing authority may lengthen this period in special cases. All spontaneous reports must be submitted immediately. Those reactions arising from clinical studies which are serious must be reported immediately whilst other minor reactions should be reported in a summary at the end of the study.

2.   Other drugs.

Spontaneous reports : Serious reactions must be reported immediately. Minor reactions need not be reported.

Clinical studies : Serious reactions must be reported immediately and this includes reactions associated with other products used in the study. Minor reactions should be reported in summary form at the end of the study.

B.   Originating from outside the UK

Serious and unpredictable reactions must be reported immediately ['unpredictable' means not previously referred to in the data sheet or the scientific literature].   Other reactions need not be reported.

MAIL 41 also stresses that companies should ensure a prompt exchange of information on adverse reactions between the parent company and subsidiaries so that this requirement can be implemented effectively.

A copy of the new standard directions sheet is included in MAIL 41.   Only the first paragraph of the previous standard direction is retained, all the remaining paragraphs being new.

Although this account summarises the new changes it is essential that any person directly involved with adverse reaction reporting in the UK should study MAIL 41 in its entirety.

I am very grateful to Mr P. Mason of the DHSS for an early copy of MAIL 41.

CHAPTER 8

A recent paper by Herman and Lorgus entitled Computer generation of the FDA-1639 form (in Clin. Res. Practices and Drug Reg. Affairs, 1983, 1, 209-225) describes the Stuart Pharmaceuticals Drug Experience Reporting System. The system uses an INQUIRE database with on-line IMS for data entry, updating and editing; the FDA-1639 form being produced by a laser printer with form design capability. Other software packages could be used for this application and output could be onto pre-printed forms rather than using an expensive laser printer.

Update

In the middle of 1984 two papers were published which dealt with premarketing safety, postmarketing safety and the ethics of the present relationship between prescribers and the industry in the U.K.

1)   M Bakke, W M Wardell and L Lasagna in a paper entitled "Commentary: Drug Discontinuation in the United Kingdom and the U.S.A. 1964 to 1983: Issues of Safety" in Clinical Pharmacology and Therapeutics Vol. 35, No. 5, P.559-567 pointed out that the U.S. system of approval, in spite of its greater restrictiveness and insistence on detail, had not proved markedly superior in preventing drugs, which were subsequently withdrawn, from going on the market.

USA regulations

The revised regulations for the United States F.D.A.'s New Drug Application Process have now been signed. ADRs must now be reported every three months for the first three years and any significant increase in side effects associated with a new drug reported immediately (Scrip No 960, Dec. 25 1984, page 16).

2)   M D Rawlins in "Doctors and the Drug Makers" in the Lancet of August 14th 1984 P.276-278 says that the charge against us (the prescribers) is that in many of our dealings with the industry we have become corrupt by accepting rewards in return for prescribing expensive products and goes on to cover many areas where the financial power of the industry is persuasive. These two articles set the scene for 1985.

U.S.A. Regulations

A revised version of the "NDA rewrite" has been published in the Federal Register on February 22 1985. This is essential reading.

Goe, and catche a falling starre,
Get with child a mandrake roote,
Tell me, where all the past yeares are
Or who cleft the divel's foot,
Teach me to heare the mermaides singing,
And to keep off envies stinging
And finde
What winde
Serves to advance an honest minde.

J. Donne

Bibliography

Drug-induced diseases, Vol. 1, 2, 3 and 4. Editor L. Meyler and H. M. Peck, Excerpta Medica, 1972

Essential reading providing background information on many different topics from an impressive list of international contributors.

Drug-induced heart disease, Vol. 5. Editor: M. R. Bristow, Elsevier, North Holland, Biomedical Press, Amsterdam, 1980

Most of the many contributors are from the U.S.A. A lot of physio-pathological detail. Well produced.

Drug Reactions and the liver. Editors: M. Davis, J. M. Tredger and R. Williams. Pitman Medical, 1981.

All the authors originate from the Liver Unit at King's College Hospital. This is an essential book with background discussion on mechanisms of ADR and the liver.

Assessing causes of adverse drug reactions. Editor: J. Venulet, Academic Press, 1982.

Based on a workshop held at Morges, Switzerland, in June 1981. Almost half the participants were Ciba-Geigy staff but with contributors from most of the world authorities. Dominated by standardised methods with few voices in opposition.

Guidelines for detection of hepatotoxicity due to drugs and chemicals. Editors: C. S. Davidson, C. M. Leevy and E.C. Chamberlayne.

U.S. Department of Health, Education and Welfare, NIH Publication No. 79-313.

An American book with all the world experts participating. This is an essential book.

Drug-induced sufferings.   Medical, pharmaceutical and legal aspects.
Editor: T. Soda, Excerpta Medica, 1980.

Proceedings of the Kyoto (Japan) International Conference against drug-
induced sufferings held in 1979.

Contributors worldwide but the majority Japanese.   Not as emotional as
the title implies.   Contains reports on most of the world ADR problems.

Monitoring for drug safety.   Editor: W. H. Inman., M.T.P. Press Ltd., 1980.

An essential book on postmarketing surveillance with a wide ranging list of
international contributors.

Meyler's Side effects of drugs, 10th edition, 1984 and the Side effects of
drugs annual, Nos.4-8 1984, Excerpta Medica.

Absolutely essential.   The most exhaustive available text on ADR of
individual drugs.

Pathology of drug-induced and toxic diseases.   Editor: R. H. Ridell,
Churchill Livingstone, 1982.

The majority of contributors are American with a sprinkling from the U.K.
Excellent, authoritative basic textbook.

Textbook of adverse drug reactions, 2nd edition.   Editor: D. M. Davies,
Oxford University Press, 1981.

Superb textbook dealing with all aspects.   Includes individual drugs, well
referenced.   Most contributors are from the north of England.

Drug-induced ocular side effects and drug interactions, 2nd edition.
Editor: F. T. Fraunfelder, Lea & Febiger, Philadelphia, 1982.

A well structured textbook on individual drugs. Based on experience of the
American National Registry of Drug-induced Ocular Side Effects.

A laboratory guide to clinical diagnosis, 5th edition.   By: R. D. Eastham;
Wright PSG, 1983.

Biochemical values in clinical medicine.   By: R. D. Eastham; John Wright
& Sons Ltd., 1978.

The subtitle is "The results following pathological or physiological change".
Both the above are excellent reference books.

A guide to drug eruptions, 3rd edition.   W. Bruinsma; De Zwaluw, P.O. Box
21, Oosthuizen, The Netherlands, 1982.

Short - 125 pages. Contains lists of drugs causing each type of skin reaction. Useful general text. Annual supplements between frequent editions.

Cutaneous side effects of systemic drugs. Editors: K. Zurcher & A. Krebs; S. Karger, Basel, 1980.

The subtitle "A commentated synopsis of today's drugs" is very accurate. Well-referenced. All text in German.

Iatrogenic diseases, 2nd edition. Editors: P. F. D'Arcy & J. P. Griffin, Oxford University Press, 1983.

Will tend to be compared with the Textbook of Adverse Drug Reactions. This has fewer contributors, all from the United Kingdom. If only one of the two was allowed, Dr. Davies' book would be the one, but I would prefer to have both since they approach the problem from different angles.

Drug monitoring. Editors: F. H. Gross & W.H.W. Inman, Academic Press, 1977.

Proceedings of an instructional workshop in Honolulu in January 1977 sponsored by Ciba-Geigy. Contributions from most of the important men in the field and now somewhat dated.

Drug monitoring. A requirement for responsible drug use. Editors: R. B. Stewart, L. E. Cluff & J. R. Philp, The Williams and Wilkins Co., Baltimore, 1977.

Most of the contributors came from Florida and describe the early American experience.

Computer aid to drug therapy and to drug monitoring. Editors: H. Ducrot, M. Goldberg, R. Hoigne & P. Middleton, North Holland Publishing Company, 1978.

Proceedings of the I.F.I.P. Working Conference of the same title, Switzerland, March 1978. The early days of computerised drug data banks.

Randomised controlled clinical trials. By: C. J. Bulpitt, Martinus Nijhoff, 1983.

One of the very few books which deals adequately with both sides of the cost/benefit ratio. Should become the standard textbook on the subject. Forms, questionnaires and the quality of life are dealt with very fully.

Immunotoxicology. Editors: G. G. Gibson, R. Hubbard & D. V. Parke, Academic Press, 1983.

The proceedings of the first international symposium on immunotoxicology in 1982. About half of its 500 pages are on drug-related topics. It is well-produced and well-referenced and has a very good chapter on drug allergy.

Adverse drug reactions: their prediction, detection and assessment. Editors: D. J. Richards & R. K. Rondel, Churchill Livingstone, 1972.

Based on a symposium organised by the Association of Medical Advisers in the Pharmaceutical Industry in 1971.   A short book (176 pages), now outdated.

Drug safety, progress and controversies.   Editors: M. Auriche, J. Burk, & J.   Duchier, Pergamon Press, 1982.

The proceedings of the IVth International Congress of Pharmaceutical Physicians, April 1981.   Largely given to adverse drug reactions and postmarketing surveillance, especially within the industry.

A manual of adverse drug interactions, 2nd edition.   Editors: J. P. Griffin & P. F. D'Arcy, John Wright & Sons Ltd., Bristol, 1979.

A good introduction to interaction mechanisms.   Interactions presented in tabulated form in pharmacological groups.   The only one with medical authors.   The first 50 pages on mechanisms and 307 pages on interactions.

Drug interactions – a source book of adverse interactions, their clinical importance, mechanisms and management.   Ivan Stockley, Blackwell Scientific Publications, 1981.

Succinct data on a large number of interactions, each dealt with individually. Easy to read. 447 pages on interactions. This book and the A.P.A. book (see below) I found easiest to read.

Evaluations of drug interactions, 2nd edition.   American Pharmaceutical Association, 2215 Constitution Avenue, N.W. Washington D.C. 20037, 1976.

Excellent monographs on individual interactions. 458 pages on interactions.

Drug interactions, 4th edition.   Editor: P. D. Hansten, Lea & Febiger, Philadelphia, 1979.

Half the book deals with drug effects on clinical laboratory results. 264 pages on interactions.

Toxicology of the eye, 2nd edition.   Editor: W. Morton Grant, Charles C. Thomas, Springfield, Illinois.

Exhaustive tome.   Covers disorders of function as well.

Paperbacks

Postmarketing surveillance of drugs.   By: L. Lasagna.   Medicine in the Public Interest Inc., 1977.

54 pages on the early American experience.

Postmarketing surveillance of adverse reactions to new medicines.   Medico-Pharmaceutical Forum, 1 Wimpole Street, London.   Publication No. 7. Report of a meeting held in December 1977.

Reflecting mainly the British approaches to the problem with an excellent paper on the practolol syndrome.

Guidelines for pre-clinical and clinical testing of new medicinal products, Part 2: Investigations in man.   A.B.P.I., 1977.

Essential basic reading.

Safety requirements for the first use of new drugs and diagnostic agents in man.   The Council for International Organisation of Medical Sciences, 1983.

Subtitled: A review of safety issues in early clinical trials of drugs. Essential reading for those involved in Phase I and II studies.

Legal and practical requirements for the registration of drugs (medicinal products) for human use, published by the International Federation of Pharmaceutical Manufacturers' Associations in Zurich 1980.   Pages 374-409 relate to postmarketing surveillance and the requirements of each nation are given in a tabular form but with little detail.

Reference volumes

Martindale.   The extra pharmacopoeia, 28th edition, 1982.   The Pharmaceutical Press, 1982.

Best source of brand names in other countries.

Pharmaceutical handbook, 19th edition.   Editor: A. Wade, The Pharmaceutical Press, London, 1980.

A companion volume to Martindale.   A Pear's Encyclopaedia of useful pharmaceutical and medical information.

Physician's desk reference, 36th edition.   Medical Economics Comp. Inc., U.S.A., 1982.

3060 pages of U.S.A. drug products.

A.B.P.I. Data Sheet Compendium, 1983-84, Datapharm Publications Ltd., 1983.

1500 pages on U.K. drug products.

Dictionnaire Vidal, 59th Edition. O.V.P., 11 rue Quentin-Bauchart, 75384, Paris.

Details of all the French drug products.

Rote Liste, Bundesverband der Pharmazeutischen Industrie, V. Karlstr. 21, 6000 Frankfurt am Main.

Details of all the German drug products.

L'informatore Farmaceutico, Organisazione Editorali, Medico-Farmaceutica S.R.L., Via Edolo 42, 20125 Milano.

Two-volume annual giving details of all Italian drug products.

Journals

Adverse drug reactions and acute poisoning reviews. Quarterly journal editied by Dr. D. M. Davies, Oxford University Press.

Excellent monographs on specific areas.

Reactions. Bi-monthly with quarterly and cummulative annual index. Adis Press, New Zealand.

Current adverse drug reaction problems.

Scrip. Editor: Dr. P. Brown, P.J.B. Publications Ltd. Published at frequent but irregular intervals.

Essential reading to find what is happening in your own company and to your own drugs, as well as the changes in the regulations and practices around the world.

Appendix

A.B.P.I. Survey (1981) of Company monitored release schemes. Completed studies

	Intended No. of patients	Actual No. of patients	Duration of treatment	Forms per patient	Rate of return of forms	Method of doctor recruitment	Intended No. of doctors	Actual	Forms returned to:	Duration of study
1	10 000	9123	0-3 months	1	Batches of 10	Reps	.-	1736	Med. Dept	2 years
2	89	89	10 days or more	1	Once	Reps	100	89	{Reg. Officer / Med. Dept.	1 year
3	6785	2944	2 years	9	9 forms/ 2 years	Reps	-	1974	Med. Dept.	3 years
4	P A S S I V E C O L L E C T I O N O F D A T A					Reps	-	-	Med. Dept.	6 months
5	201	129	12 months	11	6 x 2/12 then 3 x 3/12	Personal interview	50	42	Med. Dept.	2 years
6	50	49	9 weeks	4	On completion only	Post initially Reps latterly	-	45	Med. Dept.	19 months
7	3821	3434	5 weeks	6	After 5 weeks	Post and personal contact from Med. Dept.	600	582	Med. Dept.	18 months
8	1000	1198→994	0-3 months	5	1	Med. adviser	40	37	Med. Dept.	18 months
9	10 000	9800	6 months	6	Monthly	Reps and post	4000	-	Med. Dept.	18 months

A.B.P.I. Survey of Company monitored release schemes. Studies not yet completed

	Initial recruit-ment	Target No.	Intended duration of treatment	Target No. of forms/ patient expected	Rate of return	Method of doctor recruitment	Intended No. of doctors	Actual	Forms returned to:	Duration of study
10	25 200	17 000	1 week	3	On-going return	No Reps. Post	3500	4200	Med. Dept.	16 months
11	500	1000	2 years	4 (8-9)	3-monthly	Personal contact	-	65	Med. Dept.	3½ years
12	50	50	3 years	20	3-monthly	Direct approach	-	-	Med. Dept.	3 years
13	11 000	10 000	1 month	2	After 1 month then 6/12	Reps.	-	-	Med. Dept.	2 years
14	45	200	1-12 months	1-4 sets of forms	3-monthly	Post	-	80	Med. Dept.	2-3 years
15	1000	5000	5 years	?	Annually	Post	-	-	Med. Dept.	5 years
16	RARELY USED PRODUCT - AND EACH USE MONITORED					Lab. contacts doctor	-	-	Med. Dept.	-
17	9200	8500	3-4 months	4-7	Once at end of treatment period	Post	4000	4050	Med. Dept.	On-going
18	19 000	10 000	12 months	5	3-monthly	Reps.	9000	4500	Med. Dept.	2 years so far

CSM yellow card

IN CONFIDENCE — REPORT ON SUSPECTED ADVERSE REACTIONS

1. Please report all suspected reactions to recently introduced drugs (identified by a black triangle in the British National Formulary), vaccines, dental or surgical materials, IUCD's, absorbable sutures, contact lenses and associated fluids, and serious or unusual reactions to all agents.

2. Record all other drugs etc, including self-medication, taken in the previous 3 months. With congenital abnormalities, record all drugs taken during pregnancy, and date of last menstrual period.

3. Do not be deterred from reporting because some details are not known.

4. Please report suspected drug interactions.

NAME OF PATIENT (To allow for linkage with other reports for same patient. Please give record number for hospital patients.)	Family name					SEX	AGE or DATE OF BIRTH	WEIGHT (Kg.)
	Forenames							

DRUGS, VACCINES (Inc. Batch No.), DEVICES, MATERIALS etc. (Please give Brand Name if known)	ROUTE	DAILY DOSE	DATE		INDICATION
			STARTED	ENDED	
Suspected drug, etc.					
Other drugs, etc. (Please state if no other drug given.)					

SUSPECTED REACTIONS	STARTED	ENDED	OUTCOME (eg. fatal, recovered)

ADDITIONAL NOTES	REPORTING DOCTOR (Block letters please)
	Name:
	Address:
	Tel. No: · · · · Specialty:
	Signature: · · · · Date:

If you would like information about other reports associated with the suspected drug, please tick box —

AR/20   250,000 2/83 / 52/4286   C.BROS(N·C) Ltd.

FDA 1639

DEPARTMENT OF HEALTH AND HUMAN SERVICES PUBLIC HEALTH SERVICE FOOD AND DRUG ADMINISTRATION ROCKVILLE' MD 20857	*FORM APPROVED: OMB NO. 0910-0002* *Use of this form is prohibited after 12/31/84.*

DRUG EXPERIENCE REPORT

FDA CONTROL NO.
FDA ACCESSION NO. ☐☐☐☐☐☐☐☐☐☐☐

I. REACTION INFORMATION

1. PATIENT ID/INITIALS (In Confidence)	2. AGE	3. SEX	4. WGT.	5. HT.	6. REPORTING DATE			7. REACTION ONSET DATE		
					MO	DA	YR	MO	DA	YR

8. DESCRIBE SUSPECTED REACTION(S)

9. OUTCOME OF REACTION TO DATE
- ☐ Alive with sequelae
  - ☐ Recovered
- ☐ Still under treatment for reaction
  - ☐ Died (Give cause/date)

10. TESTS/LABORATORY DATA CONFIRMING REACTION (Include biopsy and/or autopsy results)

11. WAS OUTPATIENT TREATMENT FOR REACTION REQUIRED?
☐ Yes   ☐ No

12. WAS HOSPITAL TREATMENT FOR REACTION REQUIRED?
☐ Yes   ☐ No

II. SUSPECT DRUG(S) INFORMATION

13. SUSPECT DRUG(S) - TRADE/GENERIC NAME(S), MANUFACTURER, IND/NDA NO.	14. TOTAL DAILY DOSE
	15. ROUTE OF ADMINISTRATION

16. INDICATION(S) FOR USE	17. THERAPY DATES *(From/To)*	18. THERAPY DURATION

19a. WAS TREATMENT WITH SUSPECTED DRUG REDUCED IN DOSAGE? ☐ Yes ☐ No OR: ☐ Discontinued	19b. DID REACTION ABATE? ☐ Yes ☐ No	20a. WAS DRUG REINTRODUCED OR DOSE INCREASED? ☐ Yes ☐ No	20b. DID REACTION REAPPEAR? ☐ Yes ☐ No

III. RECENT/CONCOMITANT DRUGS AND MEDICAL PROBLEMS

21. OTHER DRUGS	TOTAL DAILY DOSE	ROUTE	DATES/DURATION OF ADMINISTRATION	INDICATIONS

22. DESCRIBE OTHER RELEVANT MEDICAL HISTORY (i.e., allergies, environmental or occupational exposure, previous drug reactions, pregnancy with gravidity/parity, ethnic origin.)

Your cooperation is needed to insure comprehensive, accurate, and timely use and interpretation of these data.

23. MFR NAME/ADDRESS	24. Check one ☐ Initial Report ☐ Follow-up Report	25. REPORTER'S NAME AND ADDRESS (In confidence)
MFR CONTROL NO. DATE SENT TO FDA		

NOTE: *Required of manufacturers by 21 CFR 310.300, 310.301 and 431.60. Manufacturers may attach additional clinical material and product analyses at their discretion.*

26. MAY THE SOURCE OF THIS REPORT BE RELEASED TO THE ARMED FORCES INSTITUTE OF PATHOLOGY? ☐ Yes ☐ No

FORM FDA 1639 (1 '82)   PREVIOUS EDITIONS ARE OBSOLETE.

FDA 1639 – reverse side

INSTRUCTIONS FOR COMPLETING FORM FDA 1639

Use a separate report form for each case. If more space is needed, additional pages may be attached.

I. Patient/Reaction Information (Items 1-12)

1. Patient ID/Initials: Record patient's identification (i.e. medical record number, initials, etc). *(This information is kept in confidence by the FDA.)*

2. Age: Record the age of the patient. When reporting a congenital malformation, record the age of the **mother**.

3. Sex: Record the sex of the patient. When reporting a congenital malformation, record the sex of the **baby.**

4. Weight: Record the weight of the patient in pounds. When reporting a congenital malformation, record the weight of the **mother.**

5. Height: Record the height of the patient in inches. When reporting a congenital malformation, record the height of the **mother.**

6. Reporting Date: Record the date when the report was initially communicated to the manufacturer.

7. Reaction Onset Date: Record the date on which the reaction was first observed or detected.

8. Suspected Reaction(s): Describe the signs, symptoms and course of the drug related event in the terminology used by the original observer of the reaction. (**Coding terms** e.g. COSTART, SNOMED, etc. may also be noted, but only **in addition** to original description.)

9. Outcome of Reaction: Indicate the status of the patient as of date indicated in Item 23. If the patient died, give the cause and date of death. Include discharge summary and/or autopsy findings, if available.

10. Tests/Laboratory Data: Describe the results of **all** diagnostic tests and exams (e.g. biochemical tests, x-rays, endoscopy, biopsy, etc.) which were done as a result of the event described in Item 8. Pertinent base line values and laboratory normals should be included with each test or exam reported. If this information is not available at the time of the initial report, a follow up report should be submitted.

11. Treatment Required: If "yes", a short description of treatment should be included in Item 8.

12. Hospitalization Required: If "yes", a short description of the treatment should be included in Item 8.

II. Suspect Drug Information (Items 13-20)

13. Suspect Drug(s): Record the trade name. The generic name should be used only when the trade name is not known. Include IND/NDA number of the drug as well as the lot number, when available.

14. Total Daily Dose: Record the total daily dose as of the date recorded in Item 7. If drug(s) was given in a different dose or form on a previous occasion, include dates and total daily dose for each drug exposure.

15. Route of Administration: Record the route of administration (i.e. po, IM, IV) as of the date recorded in Item 7.

16. Indication(s) for use: Record intended use in accepted medical terminology.

17. Therapy Dates: Give starting and stopping dates of administration for each drug listed in Item 13.

18. Therapy Duration: Give duration of therapy in days.

19. Dechallenge:
    (a) Applicable if the suspect drug(s) was either reduced in dosage or discontinued.
    (b) If 19(a) is checked, indicate whether the reaction subsided upon reduced dosage or discontinuation of the drug.

20. Rechallenge:
    (a) Applicable if the suspect drug was reintroduced to the patient's therapy after dechallenge.
    (b) If 20(a) is "yes", indicate whether or not the reaction reappeared upon rechallenge with the drug.

III. Recent/Concomitant Drugs and Medical Problems (Items 21-22)

21. List all recent or concomitant drugs. Include the total daily dose(s), indication(s) for use, route(s) of administration and dates of administration and/or duration of therapy for each drug.

22. Describe other relevant medical conditions or problems which could have contributed to the reaction. Include pertinent medical history such as allergies, occupation, industrial hazards, diet, smoking, climate, ethnic origin, cosmetics and biologicals. When reporting a congenital malformation, include the date of the last menstrual period of the mother, gravidity, parity and previous abortions.

IV. Other Information (Items 23-26)

23. Manufacturers Information: Include manufacturer's name, address, control number and date report is sent to FDA. This control number is the identifying number assigned by the manufacturer to the report for internal record control.

24. Indicate if this is an initial submission to FDA or a follow-up of a previously submitted Form FDA 1639. If this is a follow-up attach copy of initial report.

25. Record the name, title and address of the practitioner originating the report. *(This information is kept in confidence by the FDA.)*

26. Check "yes" or "no", if the source of this report may or may not be released to the Armed Forces Institute of Pathology for further study and follow-up. This is encouraged whenever possible.

Glaxo form 1 folding postage pre-paid envelope

SPACE FOR ADDITIONAL COMMENTS

Fourth Fold

Do not affix postage stamp if posted in
Gt. Britain, Channel Islands, N. Ireland
or the Isle of Man

Postage will
be paid by
Licensee

BUSINESS REPLY SERVICE
Licence No. SG 56

**Drug Surveillance Department,
Medical Division,
GLAXO GROUP RESEARCH LTD.,
WARE, HERTS. SG12 7YA**

First Fold

CONFIDENTIAL

Third Fold

Second Fold

SPACE FOR ADDITIONAL COMMENTS

Glaxo form 2

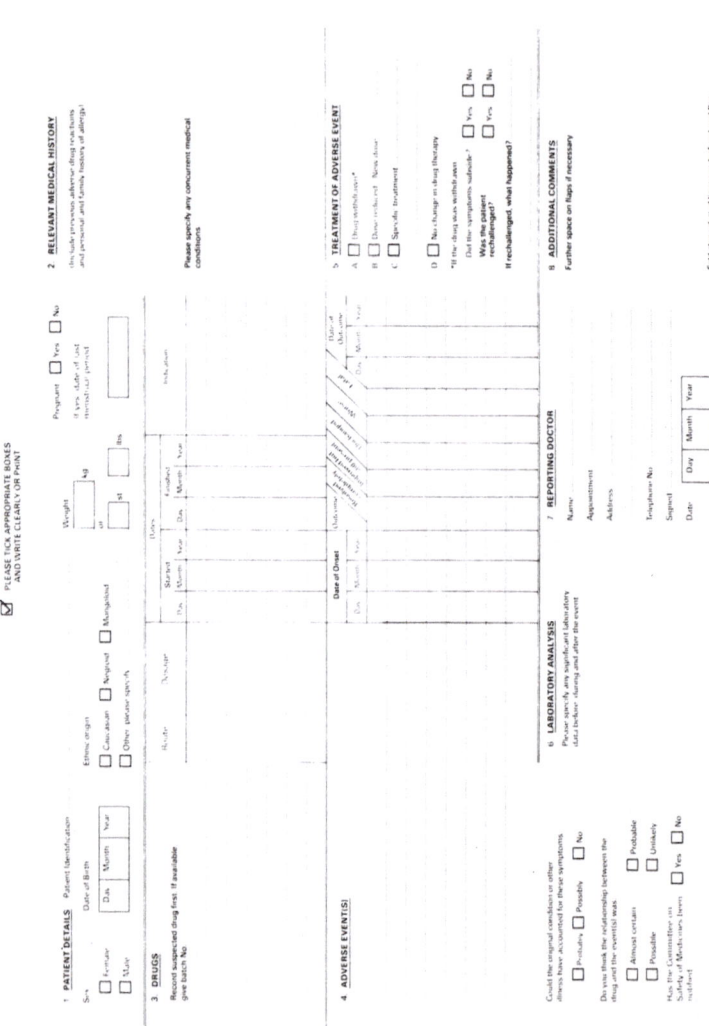

Glaxo form 2

ADVERSE EVENT REPORT FORM 2

INSTRUCTIONS

Please: 1.   Complete all sections 1-10.

2.   ☒ Mark appropriate boxes and write clearly or print.

3.   Do **not** write in any shaded areas.

4.   If space in any section is insufficient, continue
under "Additional Comments" (section 9), stating to
which section the continuation refers.

ADVERSE EVENT REPORT FORM (2)

CONFIDENTIAL

1. PATIENT DETAILS

Patient Identification: .... Hospital Number: ....

Date of Birth	Day	Month	Year

Sex ☐ Female ☐ Male

Weight ☐☐☐☐ kg.

or ☐ st. ☐ lbs.

Ethnic Origin

☐ Caucasian ☐ Negroid ☐ Mongoloid

☐ Other (please specify) ....

Was the patient?

☐ An in-patient ☐ An out-patient

☐ In general practice

☐ Other (please specify) ....

Occupation ....

Pregnant ☐ Yes ☐ No   If yes, period of gestation at time of adverse event ☐ weeks

2. MEDICAL HISTORY

Previous medical history (excluding allergy)

Current diagnoses and any concurrent medical conditions

History of Atopy ☐ Yes ☐ No

	Personal	Family
Asthma	☐	☐
Hay Fever	☐	☐
Eczema	☐	☐
Other	☐	☐

(please specify) ....

History of Allergy ☐ Yes ☐ No

If yes, please give details

Previous Adverse Drug Reactions

Drug	Reaction

3 DRUGS

DRUGS	BATCH NUMBER	ROUTE	UNIT DOSE	FREQUENCY	DATES OR TIMES						INDICATION
					STARTED			FINISHED			
					Day	Month	Year	Day	Month	Year	

Suspected drug(s)

Other drugs

4 ADVERSE EVENT(S)

ADVERSE EVENT(S)	DATE OR TIME OF ONSET			OUTCOME	PLEASE INDICATE ANY TREATMENT OF ADVERSE EVENTS
	Day	Month	Year		

RECOVERED / CONTINUING / UNCHANGED / WORSE / FATAL

DATE OF OUTCOME Day Month Year

Please continue under 'Additional Comments' if necessary

CAUSALITY

Could the original conditions have accounted for these symptoms or signs

☐ Yes ☐ Possibly ☐ No ☐ Please give details

Do you think the relationship between the drug and adverse event was

☐ Almost certain ☐ Probable ☐ Possible ☐ Unlikely

5 TREATMENT OF ADVERSE EVENTS

(a) Was the suspected drug withdrawn?

☐ Yes ☐ No

If yes

Was suspected drug withdrawn by

☐ Patient ☐ Doctor

Was the patient rechallenged with the suspected drug?

☐ Yes ☐ No

If yes, did the symptoms or signs recur?

☐ Yes ☐ No

If no

Was the dose of the suspected drug

☐ Reduced ☐ Unchanged

If reduced, new dose

(b) Did the adverse event continue?

☐ Yes ☐ No

If yes

were the symptoms or signs

☐ Considerably improved
☐ Slightly improved
☐ Unchanged
☐ Worse

Could the adverse event have continued even if the suspected drug had been withdrawn?

☐ Yes ☐ No

If no

do you think this improvement was due to

☐ Stopping suspected drug
☐ Treatment of adverse event
☐ Not known

6. RELEVANT LABORATORY FINDINGS

Please specify any significant laboratory findings before, during and after the adverse event(s)

BIOCHEMICAL AND HAEMATOLOGICAL VALUES

	Pre-treatment	1	2	3	4	Normal range		Units
Date sample taken						Lower	Upper	
Investigation	Please record values for each parameter below							

OTHER LABORATORY FINDINGS e.g. MICROBIOLOGY, URINALYSIS

	Pre-treatment	1	2	3	4	5
Date sample taken						
Investigation	Please record values for each parameter below					

| A | E | Type | Variant | New? | Record No. |

7. BIOPSY AND/OR POST MORTEM RESULTS

Was a biopsy performed?   ☐ Yes   ☐ No

| Day | Month | Year |

If yes, please give date
and details..
....

Special

12 | I | | 14

15 | | | | | 19

Lab. codes

20 | | | | | 23

24 | | | | | 27

28 | | | | | 31

32 | | | | | 35

36 | | | | | 39

40 | | | | | 43

44 | | | | | 47

48 | | | | | 51

52 | | | | | 55

56 | | | | | 59

60 | | | | | 63

64 | | | | | 67

If the patient died, was a post mortem performed?   ☐ Yes   ☐ No

| Day | Month | Year |

If yes, please give date of death

and post mortem details (preferably copy of post mortem report)
....

8. SPECIALIST OPINION

Was a further specialist opinion sought?   ☐ Yes   ☐ No

| Day | Month | Year |

If yes, please give date

Name of specialist..

Appointment ....

Opinion ....
....

Report

12 | J | | 14

15 | | | | | 19

Lab. codes

20 | | | | | 23

24 | | | | | 27

28 | | | | | 31

32 | | | | | 35

36 | | | | | 39

40 | | | | | 43

44 | | | | | 47

48 | | | | | 51

52 | | | | | 55

56 | | | | | 59

60 | | | | | 63

9. ADDITIONAL COMMENTS

Have you notified your drug regulatory authority (e.g. F.D.A., C.S.M.)?   ☐ Yes   ☐ No

10. REPORTING DOCTOR

Name...

Appointment...

Address..
....

Country................................. Telephone No...........................

Signature...

| Day | Month | Year |

Glaxo adverse skin reaction form

ADVERSE SKIN REACTION REPORT FORM

INSTRUCTIONS

Please: 1. Complete all sections 1-10.

2. $\boxed{\text{X}}$ Mark appropriate boxes and write clearly or print.

3. Do **not** write in any shaded areas.

4. If space in any section is insufficient, continue under "Additional Comments" (section 9), stating to which section the continuation refers.

ADVERSE SKIN REACTION FORM

CONFIDENTIAL

1. PATIENT DETAILS

Patient Identification:... Hospital Number:..

Date of Birth	Day	Month	Year

Sex ☐ Female ☐ Male

Weight ☐☐☐☐☐☐ kg.

or ☐ st. ☐ lbs.

Ethnic Origin

☐ Caucasian ☐ Negroid ☐ Mongoloid

☐ Other (please specify).............................

Was the patient?

☐ An in-patient ☐ An out-patient

☐ In general practice

☐ Other (please specify)...........................

Occupation ....

Pregnant ☐ Yes ☐ No   If yes, period of gestation at time of adverse event ☐ weeks

2. MEDICAL HISTORY

Previous medical history (excluding allergy)

Current diagnoses and any concurrent conditions

History of Atopy ☐ Yes ☐ No

	Personal	Family
Asthma	☐	☐
Hay Fever	☐	☐
Eczema	☐	☐
Other	☐	☐

(please specify)...

History of Allergy ☐ Yes ☐ No

If yes, please give details

Previous Adverse Drug Reactions

Drug	Reaction
....	....
....	....
....	....
....	....

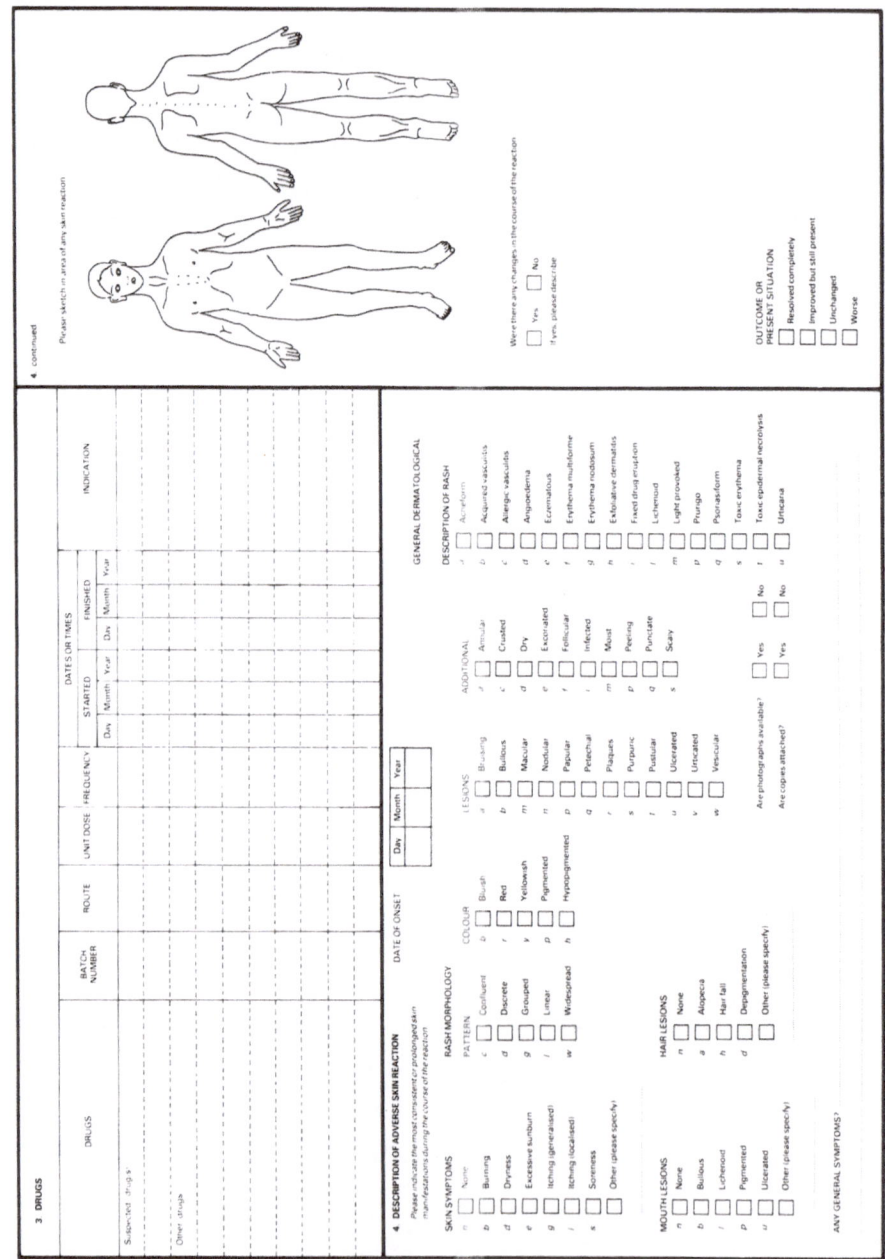

5. MANAGEMENT OF ADVERSE REACTION

(a) Was the suspected drug withdrawn?

☐ Yes   ☐ No

If yes

Was suspected drug withdrawn by

☐ Patient   ☐ Doctor

Was the patient rechallenged with the suspected drug?

☐ Yes   ☐ No

If yes, did the symptoms or signs recur?

☐ Yes   ☐ No

Treatment of adverse reaction

....
....
....
....

If no

Was the dose of the suspected drug

☐ Reduced   ☐ Unchanged

If reduced, new dose...........................

(b) Did the adverse event continue?

☐ Yes   ☐ No

If yes

were the symptoms or signs

☐ Considerably improved
☐ Slightly improved
☐ Unchanged
☐ Worse

Could the adverse event have continued even if the suspected drug had been withdrawn?

☐ Yes   ☐ No

If no

do you think this improvement was due to:

☐ Stopping suspected drug
☐ Treatment of adverse reaction
☐ Not known

6. INVESTIGATION OF ADVERSE REACTION

SKIN TESTS   Results

	Yes	No	Positive	Negative
Patch tests	☐	☐	☐	☐ ....
Prick test	☐	☐	☐	☐ ....
Intra-dermal test	☐	☐	☐	☐ ....
Biopsy of a lesion	☐	☐		....
Immunofluorescence of a lesion	☐	☐		....

Other (please specify)...

7. CASUAL RELATIONSHIP

Could the original conditions or other illnesses have accounted for this skin reaction?

☐ Yes   ☐ Possibly   ☐ No   Please give details...
....

Do you think the relationship between the drug and adverse event was

☐ Almost certain   ☐ Probable   ☐ Possible   ☐ Unlikely

Type Variant New? Record No.

A E

Special

12 I 14

15 | | | | 19

Lab codes

20 | | | | 23

24 | | | | 27

28 | | | | 31

32 | | | | 35

36 | | | | 39

40 | | | | 43

44 | | | | 47

48 | | | | 51

52 | | | | 55

56 | | | | 59

60 | | | | 63

64 | | | | 67

Report

12 J 14

15 | | | | 19

Lab codes

20 | | | | 23

24 | | | | 27

28 | | | | 31

32 | | | | 35

36 | | | | 39

40 | | | | 43

44 | | | | 47

48 | | | | 51

52 | | | | 55

56 | | | | 59

60 | | | | 63

8. RELEVANT LABORATORY FINDINGS

Please specify any significant laboratory findings before, during and after the adverse skin reaction.

9. SPECIALIST OPINION

Was a further specialist opinion sought?   ☐ Yes   ☐ No

Day	Month	Year

If yes, please give date*

Name of specialist...

Appointment ....

Opinion ....

....

....

10. ADDITIONAL COMMENTS

Have you notified your drug regulatory authority (e.g. F.D.A., C.S.M.)?   ☐ Yes   ☐ No

11. REPORTING DOCTOR

Name ....

Appointment ....

Address...

....

Country...................................... Telephone No. ....

Signature............ ....

Day	Month	Year

Wellcome Research Laboratories ADR transcription forms

ADVERSE EXPERIENCE CODING FORM, C.C.O. C.R.D.

Card 1 — Date of Reaction — Drug — Race — Age — Sex — Pregnant — LMP — File No. — Date — Rec'd. Yr/Mth/Day

Card 2 — No. of Patients — Country — Yr/Mth/Day — Doctor's Name

Card 3 — Drug Form — Strength (Mg) — Daily Dose — Duration

Card 4 — 2nd Drug — Route — Daily Dose — Duration

Card 4 — 3rd Drug — Route — Daily Dose — Duration

Card 4 — 4th Drug — Route — Daily Dose — Duration

Card 4 — 5th Drug — Route — Daily Dose — Duration

Card 4 — 6th Drug — Route — Daily Dose — Duration

WELLCOME HANDWRITING CONVENTION	
1=figure one	1=letter 'EYE'
7=figure seven	5=letter 'ESS'
0=zero	Z=letter 'ZED'
0=space	0=letter 'OH'

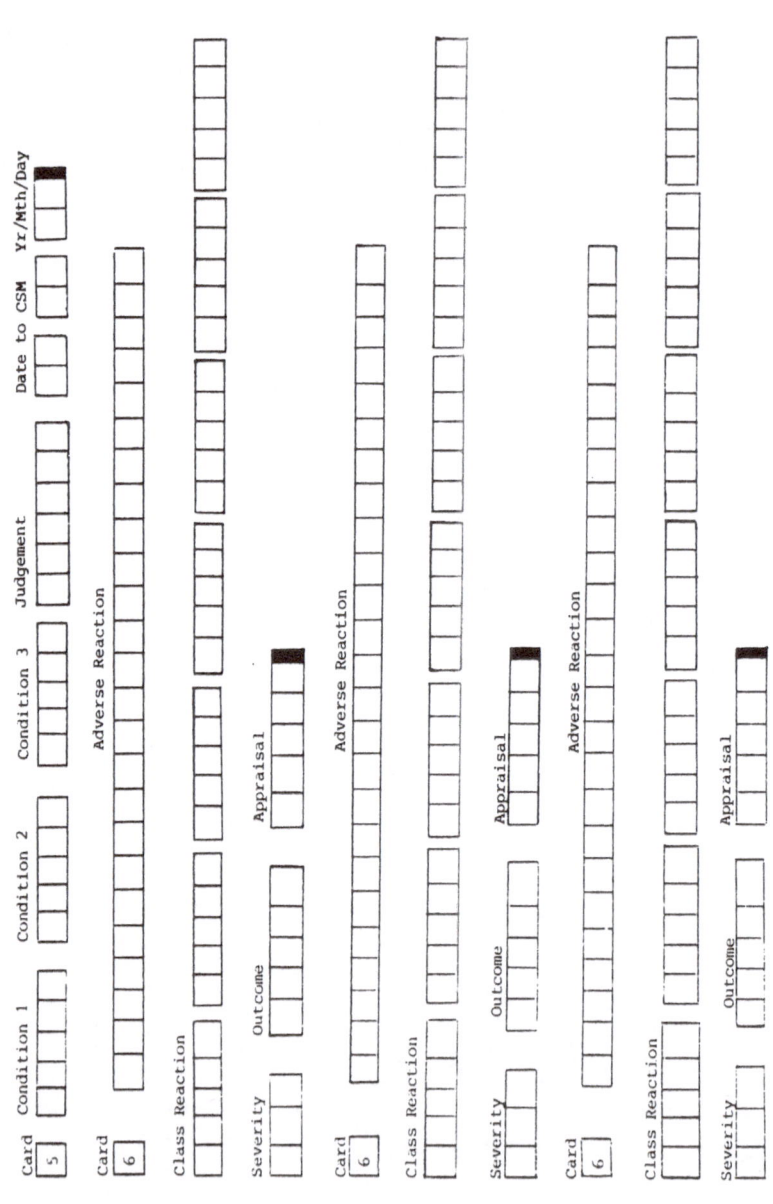

Card
6

Class Reaction

Adverse Reaction

Severity

Outcome

Appraisal

Card
6

Class Reaction

Adverse Reaction

Severity

Outcome

Appraisal

Card
6

Class Reaction

Adverse Reaction

Severity

Outcome

Appraisal

UNCONTROLLED CLINICAL TRIAL ADVERSE EVENT FORM

Acute
treatment

Important. Please enter the appropriate patient number before returning book ⟶

PATIENT'S TRIAL No.

TRIAL   **ADVERSE EVENT FORM**

Date

Patient's name ....

Please insert 'x' where appropriate   Physician's name ....

ADVERSE EVENT(S)	Date of onset			Outcome	Resolved completely	Improved but still present	Unchanged	Worse	Fatal	Date of outcome		
	Day	Month	Year							Day	Month	Year
1.												
2.												
3.												
4.												

TREATMENT OF ADVERSE EVENT(S)

A ☐   Trial drug withdrawn*

B ☐   Trial dose reduced: if so, please state new dose: ....

C ☐   Specific treatment (please specify): ....

....

D ☐   No change in trial drug therapy

* If the trial drug was withdrawn:

Did the symptoms subside?   Yes ☐   No ☐

Was the patient re-challenged?   Yes ☐   No ☐

If 'yes', what happened? : ....

....

RELEVANT MEDICAL HISTORY

Please specify any previous adverse reactions and personal or family history of allergy : ....

....

....

Please specify concurrent medication (dose and frequency): ....

....

....

Could the patient's original condition or other illness account for the adverse event?

       Yes ☐   Possibly ☐   No ☐

Do you think the relationship between the trial drug and the adverse event was

Almost certain ☐   Probable ☐   Possible ☐   Unlikely ☐

Investigator's Signature ....

MINOR ADVERSE EVENTS FORM

INSTRUCTIONS

Complete this form for minor adverse events.

Go to Major Adverse Event Form if:

1. Study drug has been discontinued
2. If you consider the event to be serious or life-threatening
3. The patient has died (any cause)
4. If a clinical diagnosis has been made

TRIAL No.   **VISIT**

ADVERSE EVENT(S) Please give full description including duration, frequency and severity. Use a new line for each separate event.	Date of onset			Outcome Resolved completely / Improved but still present / Unchanged / Worse				Date of outcome			Causality (see below)
	Day	Month	Year					Day	Month	Year	

If adverse event developed within the first 24 hours,
please give time to onset in hours ....

Causality – please indicate above your opinion of the relationship between study drug and event as follows:

1. Unlikely
2. Possible
3. Probable
4. Almost certain

Treatment of Adverse Event   ☐ Yes   ☐ No

If you, please specify, with dose, frequency and duration of treatment:

....
....
....
....

Physician's signature: ....Date: ....

If it should become necessary to stop treatment, please fill in Major Events Form.

MAJOR ADVERSE EVENTS FORM

Please complete as soon as possible after adverse event and return immediately to address overleaf.

1. PATIENT DETAILS

TRIAL No

Weight

kg

or

st   lbs

Date of Birth

☐ Female
☐ Male

Day	Month	Year

Ethnic origin

☐ Caucasian   ☐ Negroid   ☐ Mongoloid

☐ Other (please specify)

2. RELEVANT MEDICAL HISTORY
(Include previous adverse drug reactions and personal and family history of allergy)

3. DRUGS

Study drug:

Other drugs:

	Route	Daily dosage	Dates						Indication
			Started			Finished			
			Day	Month	Year	Day	Month	Year	

4. ADVERSE EVENT(S)
Please describe event, its severity and all symptoms

	Date of onset			Outcome						Date of outcome		
	Day	Month	Year	Resolved completely	Improved but still present	Unchanged	Worse	Fatal		Day	Month	Year

5. TREATMENT OF ADVERSE EVENT

A ☐ Drug withdrawn*
B ☐ Dose reduced. New dose: _____
C ☐ Specific treatment: _____

D ☐ No change in drug therapy.

*If the drug was withdrawn:

Did the symptoms subside?   ☐ Yes   ☐ No

Was the patient rechallenged?   ☐ Yes   ☐ No

If rechallenged, what happened? _____

Could the original condition or other illness have accounted for these symptoms:

☐ Probably   ☐ Possibly   ☐ No

Do you think the relationship between the drug and the event(s) was:

☐ Almost certain   ☐ Probable
☐ Possible   ☐ Unlikely

7. REPORTING DOCTOR

Name: _____

Address: _____

Telephone No: _____

Signed: _____

Date:

Day	Month	Year

6. LABORATORY ANALYSIS
Please specify any significant laboratory data before, during and after the event overleaf

8. ADDITIONAL COMMENTS   overleaf

Pre-marketing clinical trials compared with post-marketing surveillance schemes

		P.M.C.T.	P.M.S. Schemes
1.	Numbers involved	1000 to 3000	100 to 30,000
2.	Efficiency of reporting	Probably better than 95% of ADR	Variable
3.	Patient drop-outs	Few	Many
4.	Intervening diseases	Responsibility for diagnosis of serious intervening disease retained by trialist	Responsibility for diagnosis of serious intervening disease passed to hospital service
5.	Regulatory authorities	Mandatory interest	?Less interest - sometimes very little
6.	Pharmaceutical company	Mandatory interest	?Less interest - sometimes very little
7.	Routine laboratory investigations	Yes	Rarely and then usually less intensive
8.	Publication	Routine, usually top journals	50% published, rarely top journals
9.	Staff	Usually hand-picked hospital staff consultants	General practitioners - often selected by company responsible
10.	Duration	Usually short term	Variable: short to long term
11.	Professional interest of doctors	Very high	Low
12.	Documentation	Must satisfy regulatory authorities	Minimal
13.	Controls	Majority of patients in randomised controlled studies	Controls rare; randomised never
14.	Patients	Narrow criteria of entry	Wide criteria of entry
15.	Allocation of staff from pharmaceutical company per patient	High	Low
16.	Statistical evaluation	Common	Rare
17.	Results quoted in advertisements	Always	?Never
18.	Background incidence of other disease	Low	High
19.	Seeding value	Low	High
20.	Patient assessment	Mostly objective	Mostly subjective

Working causality algorithm for drug-event associations
(from Dr A. Ruskin)

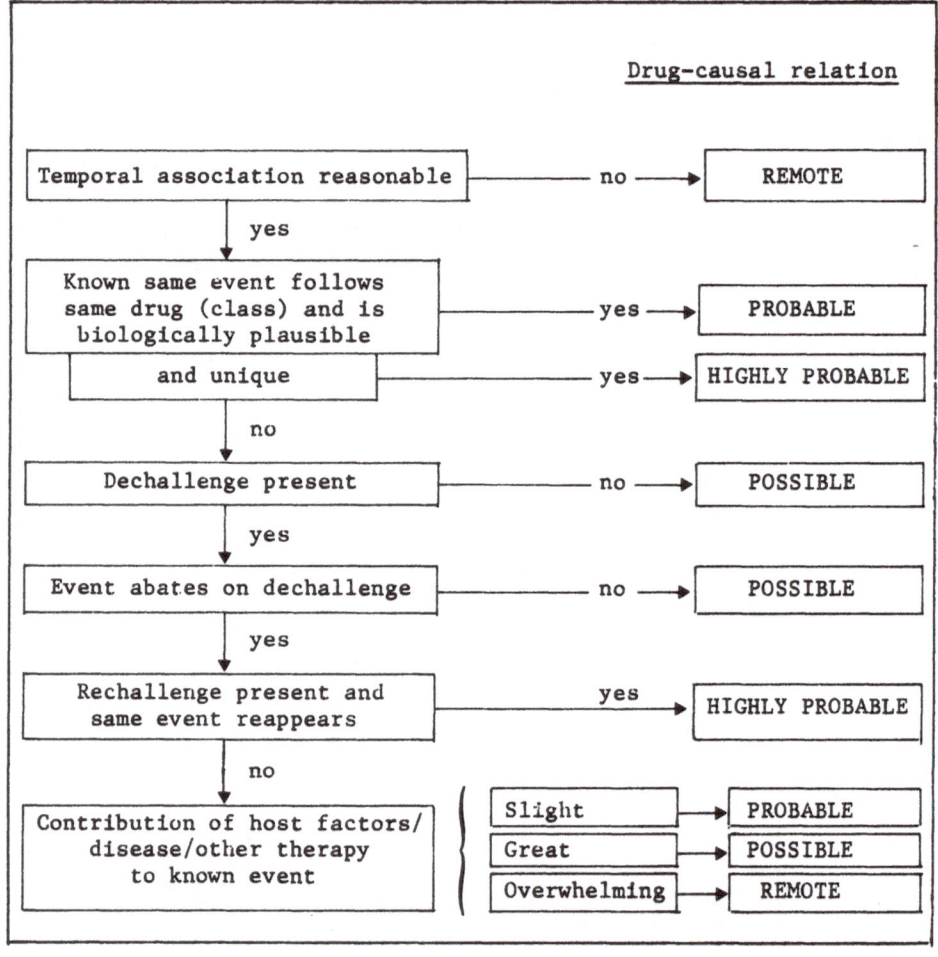

Working causality algorithm for drug-death associations
(from Dr A. Ruskin)

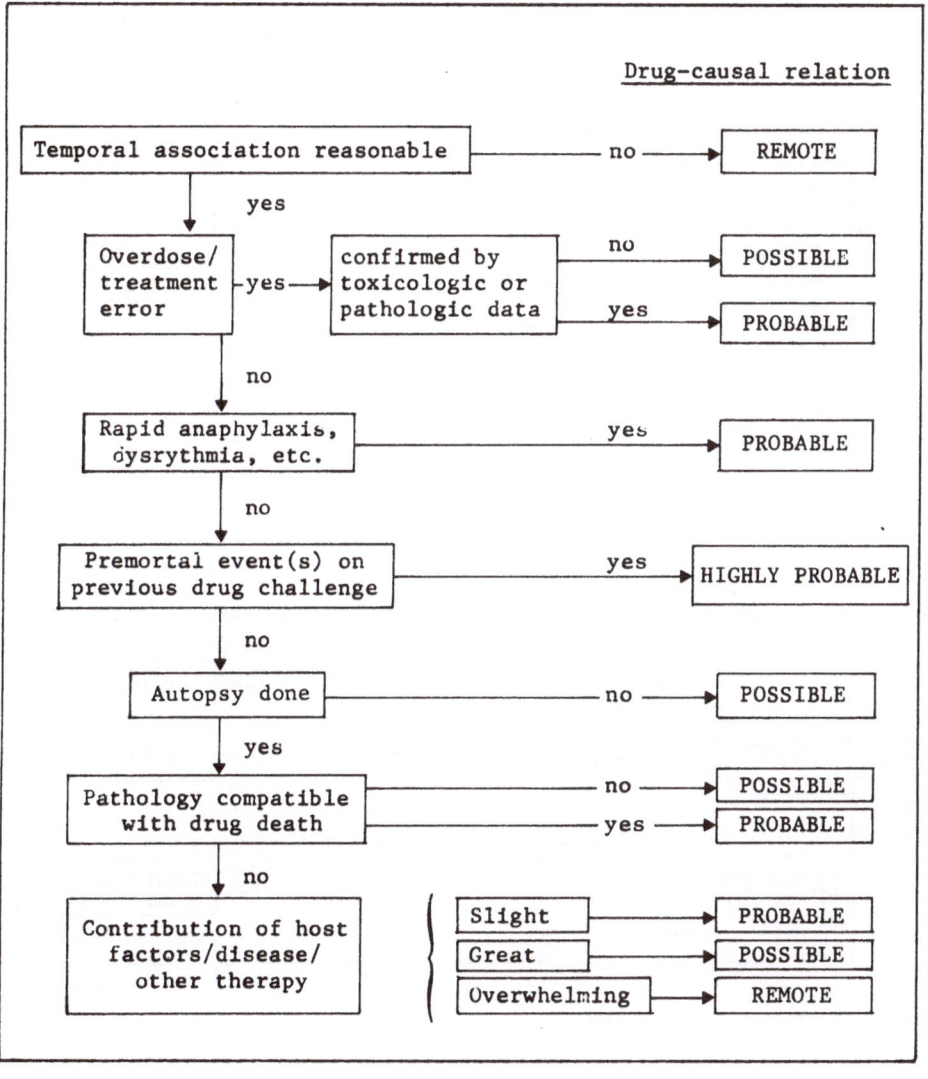

Algorithm for assessing causal relationship between drug and
event; August 1983 Revision (A. Emanueli, Farmitalia Carlo Erba,
Milan, Italy)

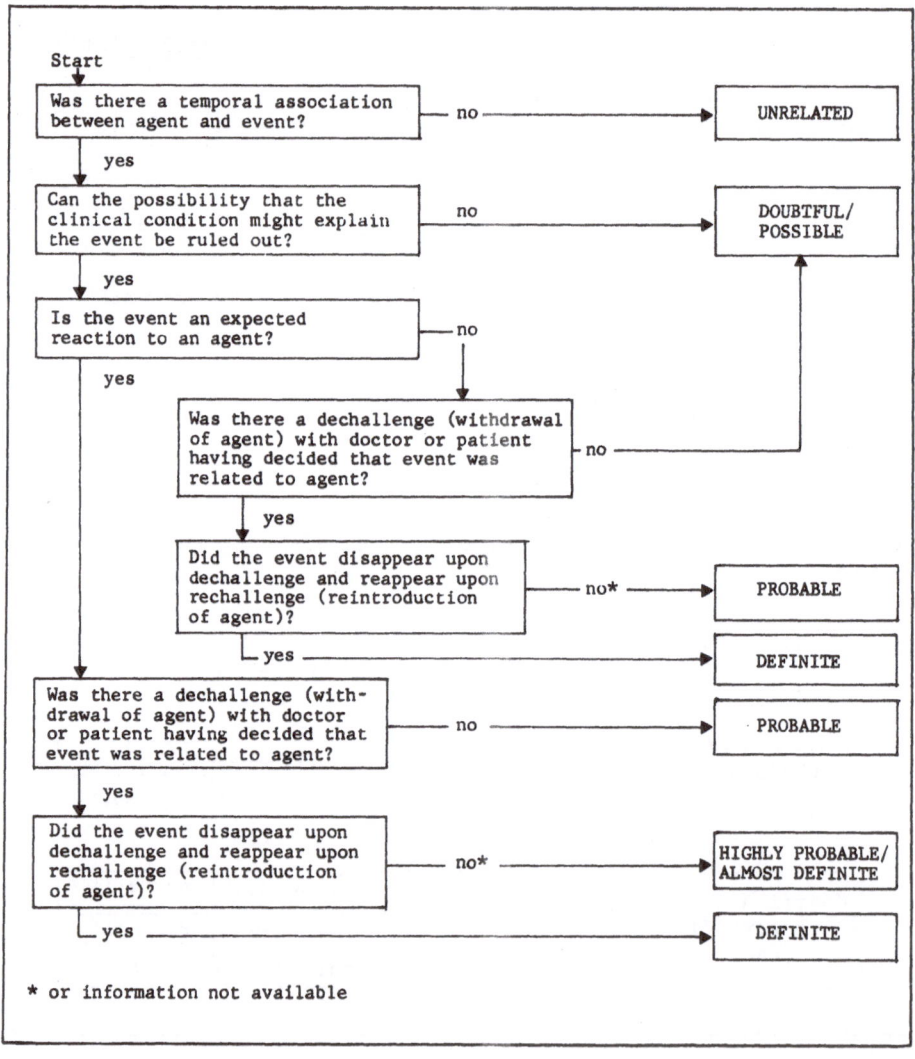

References

Chapter 1

1. Distillers Company (Biochemicals Ltd). Distaval. Lancet, 1961, 2, 1262
2. Nicholls, J.J. The Practolol Syndrome - a retrospective analysis. In Post-marketing Surveillance of Adverse Reactions to New Medicines. Medico-pharmaceutical Forum, Publication No. 7, 1977
3. Anon. Thalidomide's long shadow. Br. Med. J., 1976, 2, 1155
4. Skegg, D.C.G. and Doll, R. The case for recording events in clinical trials. Br. Med. J., 1977, 2, 1523-1524
5. Hemminki, L. Study of information submitted by drug companies to licensing authorities. Br. Med. J., 1980, 1, 836
6. Skegg, D.C.G. Adverse reaction monitoring in the future. In Pharmaceutical Medicine (ed. N. Macleod), Churchill Livingstone, 1979, p.144
7. Dollery, C.T. Clinical trials of new drugs. J. R. Coll. Physicians Lond., 1977, 11 (3), 226-233
8. Inman, W.H.W. Monitoring by voluntary reporting at national level. In Adverse Drug Reactions (ed. D.J. Richards and R.K. Rondel), Churchill Livingstone, 1972
9. Inman, W.H.W. and Adelstein, A.M. Rise and fall of asthma mortality in England and Wales in relation to pressurised aerosols. Lancet, 1969, 2, 279
10. Crooks, J. The detection of adverse drug reactions. J. R. Coll. Physicians Lond., 1977, 11 (3), 239-244
11. Tierney, S. The testing of new drugs and the responsibility for their unforeseen effects. J. R. Coll. Physicians Lond., 1977, 11 (3), 237
12. Beral, V. et al. Mortality among oral contraceptive users. Lancet, 1977, 2, 727-731
13. Bader, J.-P. Scrip, 1981, No. 639, 1
14. Schönhöfer, P. Scrip, 1981, No. 638, 2
15. Melmon, K.L. and Nierenberg, D.W. Drug interactions and the prepared observer. New Engl. J. Med., 1981, 304 (12), 723-725

16. Wright, P. Untoward effects associated with Practolol administration: oculomucocutaneous syndrome. Br. Med. J., 1975, 1, 595-598.

17. Herbst, A.L., Ulfelder, H. and Poskager, D.C. Association of maternal stilboestrol therapy with tumour appearance in young women. New Engl. J. Med., 1971, 284, 891

18. Committee of Principal Investigators. A co-operative trial in the primary prevention of ischaemic heart disease using clofibrate. Br. Heart J., 1978, 40, 1069-1118

19. Committee of Principal Investigators. WHO co-operative trial on primary prevention of ischaemic heart disease using clofibrate to lower serum cholesterol: Mortality follow-up. Lancet, 1980, 2, 379-385

20. Cross, K.W. Cost of preventing retrolental fibroplasia. Lancet, 1973, 2, 954-956.

21. Bolton, D.P.G. and Cross, K.W. Further observations on cost of preventing retrolental fibroplasia. Lancet, 1974, 1, 445-458

22. Miller, D.L., Ross, E.M., Alderslade, R., Bellman, M.H. and Rawson, N.S.B. Pertussis immunisation and serious acute neurological illness in children. Br. Med. J., 1981, 282 (6276), 1565

23. Meade, T.W. Pertussis vaccine. Br. Med. J., 1981, 283, 59

24. Anon. Pertussis vaccine. Br. Med. J., 1981, 282 (6276), 1563-1564

25. Fleming, D.M., Knox, J.D.E. and Crombie, D.L. Debendox in early pregnancy and fetal malformation. Br. Med. J., 1981, 283, 99-101

26. Dinman, B.D. Occupational health and the reality of risk - an eternal dilemma of tragic choice. J. Occup. Med., 1980, 22 (3), 153-157

27. Dinman, B.D. The reality and acceptance of risk. J.A.M.A., 1980, 244 (11), 1226-1228

28. Daily Telegraph. 3 June 1981 - 25 June 1981

29. Pochin, E.E. The acceptance of risk. Br. Med. Bull., 1975, 184

30. Porter, J. and Jick, H. Drug-related deaths among medical in-patients. J.A.M.A., 1977, 237, 879

31. Girdwood, R.H. Deaths after taking medicaments. Br. Med. J., 1974, 1, 501-504

32. Anon. Hunting rare adverse drug reactions. Br. Med. J., 1981, 282 (6261), 342

33. Inman, W.H.W. Postmarketing surveillance of adverse drug reactions in general practice, I. Br. Med. J., 1981, 282, 1131-1132

34. Shapiro, S. Postmarketing assessment of drugs. In Post-marketing Surveillance of Adverse Reactions to New Medicines. Medico-pharmaceutical Forum, Publication No. 7, 1977

35. Lewis, J.A. Postmarketing surveillance: How many patients? Trends Pharmacol. Sci., 1981, 2 (4), 93-94

36. Anon. Rauwolfia and breast cancer. Lancet, 1975, 2, 312

37. Spriet-Pourra, C., Spriet, A., Soubrie, C. and Simon, P. Les méthodes d'étude des effets indésirables des médicaments, II: Thérapie, 1982, **37**, 13-22
38. Finney, D.J. The design and logic of a monitor of drug use. J. Chron. Dis., 1965, **18**, 77
39. Inman, W.H.W. Postmarketing surveillance of adverse drug reactions in general practice, II. Br. Med. J., 1981, **282** (6271), 1216-1217
40. Karch, F.E. and Lasagna, L. Adverse drug reactions. J.A.M.A., 1975, **234** (12), 1236
41. Division of Drug Experience, Food and Drug Administration. Procedural Manual for Handling Drug Experience Reports. Glossary, Paper flow and Algorithms, 1980
42. Kramer, M.S., Leventhal, J.M., Hutchinson, T.A. and Feinstein, A.R. An algorithm for the operational assessment of adverse drug reactions, I: Background, description for use and instruction. J.A.M.A., 1979, **242** (7), 623-632
43. Weintraub, M. Recording events in clinical trials. Br. Med. J., 1978, **i**, 581
44. Simpson, R.J., Tiplady, B. and Skegg, D.C.G. Event recording in a clinical trial of a new medicine. Br. Med. J., 1980, **280**, 1133-1134
45. Anon. Lessons from the Benoxaprofen affair. Lancet, 1982, Sept. 4, 529
46. Seventh European Symposium on Clinical Pharmacological Evaluation in Drug Control. W.H.O. Euro Reports and Studies, 13
47. Rawlins, M.D. and Thompson, J.W. Pathogenesis of adverse drug reactions. In Textbook of Adverse Drug Reactions (ed. D.M. Davies), Oxford University Press, 1977, pp.10-31
48. Venulet, J. Monitoring adverse reactions to drugs. In Progress in Drug Research (ed. E. Jucken), Berghausen Verlag, Basle, 1977
49. Bennett, B.S. and Lipman, A.G. Comparative study of prospective surveillance and voluntary reporting in determining the incidence of adverse drug reactions. Am. J. Hosp. Pharm., 1977, **34**, 931-936
50. Reidenberg, M.M. and Lowenthal, D.J. Adverse non-drug reactions. New Engl. J. Med., 1968, **279** (13), 678-679
51. Bulpitt, C.J., Dollery, C.T. and Carne, S. A symptom questionnaire for hypertensive patients. J. Chron. Dis., 1974, **27**, 309-323
52. Bulpitt, C.J., Dollery, C.T. and Carne, S. Change in symptoms of hypertensive patients after referral to hospital clinic. Br. Heart J., 1976, **38**, 121-128
53. Joubert, P.H., Van Rijssen, F.W.J. and Venter, J.P. Drug side effects assessed in a 'naturalistic' setting. S. Afr. Med. J., 1977, **52**, 34-36
54. Joyce, C.R.B. Placebos and other comparative treatments. Br. J. Clin. Pharmacol., 1982, **13**, 313-318
55. Pogge, R.C. The toxic placebo. Med. Times, 1965, **91** (8), 773-776

56. Wolf, S. Placebos. Ass. Res. Nerv. Dis. Proc., 1959, 37

57. Wolf, S. Effects of suggestion and conditioning on the action of chemical agents in human subjects: the pharmacology of placebos. J. Clin. Invest., 1950, 29, 100

58. Wolf, S. and Pinsky, R.H. Effects of placebo administration and occurrence of toxic reactions. J.A.M.A., 1954, 155 (4), 339-341

59. Vinar, O. Dependence on a placebo: a case report. Br. J. Psychiat., 1969, 115, 1189-1190

60. Domecq, C., Naranjo, C.A., Ruiz, I. and Busto, U. Sex-related variations in the frequency and characteristics of adverse drug reactions. J. Clin. Pharmacol. Ther. Toxicol., 1980, 18 (8), 362-366

61. Green, D.M. Pre-existing conditions, placebo reactions and 'side effects'. Ann. Intern. Med., 1964, 60 (2), 255-265

62. Letemendia, F.J.J. and Harris, A.D. The influence of side effects on the reporting of symptoms. Psychopharmacologia, 1959, 1, 39-47

63. Wolf, S. The pharmacology of placebo. Pharmacol. Rev., 1959, 11, 689

64. Tucker, W.B. Effects of placebo administration and occurrence of toxic reactions. J.A.M.A., 1954, 155, 339

65. Thompson, R. Side effects and placebo amplification. Br. J. Psychiat., 1982, 140, 64-68

66. Lasagna, L., Mosteller, F., Von Felsinger, J.M. and Beecher, H.K. A study of placebo response. Am. J. Med., 1954, June, 770-779

67. Knowles, J.B. and Lucas, C.J. Experimental studies of the placebo response. J. Ment. Sci., 1960, 106, 231-240

68. Beecher, H.K. The powerful placebo. J.A.M.A., 1955, 2 Dec., 1602-1606

69. Lasagna, L., Laties, V.G. and Dohan, J.L. Further studies on the 'pharmacology' of placebo administration. J. Clin. Invest., 1958, 37, 533-537

70. Fields, H.L. and Levine, J.D. Biology of placebo analgesia. Am. J. Med., 1981, 70 (4), 745-746

71. Levine, J.D., Gordon, N.C. and Fields, H.L. The mechanism of placebo analgesia. Lancet, 1978, 23 Sept., 654-657

72. Norwegian Multicenter Study Group. Timolol-induced reduction in mortality and reinfarction in patients surviving acute myocardial infarction. New Engl. J. Med., 1981, 34 (14), 801-807

73. Schindel, L. Placebo-induced side effects. In Drug Induced Diseases (ed. L. Meyler and H.M. Peck), Excerpta Medica, Amsterdam

Chapter 2

74. Petrie, W.M. and Levine, J. The assessment of adverse reactions in clinical trials. Int. Pharmacopsychiat., 1978, 13, 209-216

75. Inman, W.H.W. The United Kingdom. In Monitoring for Drug Safety, M.T.P. Press, 1980

76. Gau, D.W. and Diehl, A.K. Disagreement among general practitioners regarding cause of death. Br. Med. J., 1982, 284, 239-242

77. Cameron, H.M. and McGregor, E. Prospective study of 1152 hospital autopsies, 1: Inaccuracies in death certification. J. Pathol., 1981, 133, 273-283

78. Harlow, B.J. Monitoring of adverse reactions by a pharmaceutical company before marketing. In Adverse Drug Reactions (ed. D.J. Richards and R.K. Rondel), Churchill Livingstone, 1972

79. Downing, R.W., Rickets, K. and Meyers, F. Side reactions in neurotics, I: A comparison of two methods of assessment. J. Clin. Pharmacol., 1970, Sept-Oct., 289-297

80. Bulpitt, C.J. Randomised Controlled Clinical Trials, Martinus Nijhoff, The Hague, 1983

81. Bulpitt, C.J., Dollery, C.T. and Carne, S. A symptom questionnaire for hypertensive patients. J. Chron. Dis., 1974, 27, 309-323

82. Howie, J.G.R. and Clark, G.A. Double blind trial of early demethylchlortetracycline in minor respiratory illness in general practice. Lancet, 1970, 2, 1009

83. Laferrière, N., Tenaillon, A., Saltiel, J.C., Smagghe, A., Chicon, F.J., Chretien, J. and Portos, J.L. Le questionnaire médical 1978, INSERM, Paris, 1977

84. Bond, A. and Lader, M. The use of analogue scales in rating subjective feelings. Br. J. Med. Psychol., 1974, 47, 211-218

85. Aitken, R.C.B. Measurement of feelings using analogue scales. Proc. R. Soc. Med., 1969, 62, 989-993

86. Huskisson, E.C. Assessment for clinical trials. Clin. Rheumat. Dis., 1976, 2 (1), 37-49

87. McGavin, C.R., Artvinli, M., Nave, M. and McHardy, G.J.R. Dyspnoea, disability and distance walked. Comparison of estimates of exercise performance in respiratory disease. Br. Med. J., 1978, 2, 241-243

88. Zealley, A.K. and Aitken, C.B. Measurement of mood. Proc. R. Soc. Med., 1969, 62, 993-996

89. Glaser, E.M. Volunteers, controls, placebos and questionnaires in clinical trials. In Medical Surveys and Clinical Trials (ed. L.J. Witts), Oxford Medical, 1964

90. Beck, A.T., Ward, C.M., Mendelsohn, M., Mock, J. and Erbaugh, J. An inventory for measuring depression. Arch. Gen. Psychiat., 1961, 4, 561-571

91. Hamilton, M.A. A rating scale for depression. J. Neurol. Neurosurg. Psychiat., 1960, 23, 56

92. US Department of Health, Education and Welfare Alcohol, Drug Abuse and Mental Health Administration. Dotes. Dosage Record and Treatment Emergent Symptom Scale. In ECDEU Assessment Manual, p.223-245

93. Vinar, O. Scale for rating treatment emergent symptoms in psychiatry. Act. Nerv. Sup., 1971, 238-240

94. SAFTEE. A new method for assessing side effects in clinical trials. Cont. Clin. Trials, 1983, **4**, 157

95. Anderson, K., Malm, U., Perris, C., Rapp, W. and Roman, G. The inter-rater reliability of scales for rating symptoms and side effects in schizophrenia patients during a clinical trial. Acta.Psychiat. Scand. Suppl., 1974, **249**, 38-42

96. Gagnon, M.A. and Tebreault, L. Pharmacologie humaine des anorexigénes. Validité d'un questionnaire sur l'appetit. Un Med. Can., Vol. **104**, Juin 1975, p.922-929

97. Pearson, R.G. and Byars, G.E. The development and validation of a checklist for measuring subjective fatigue. School of Aviation Medicine, USAF Report No. 56-115, 1956

98. Avery, C.W., Bertram, P.I., Allison, B. and Mandell, N. Systematic errors in the evaluation of side effects. Am. J. Psychiat., 1967, **123** (Jan.), 875-878

99. Downing, R.W., Rickets, K. and Meyers, F. Side reactions in neurotics: a comparison of two methods of assessment. J. Clin. Pharmacol., 1970, Sept-Oct., 289-297

100. Lapierre, Y.D. Evaluation des effets secondaires chez les neurotiques. Un essai avec les mésoridazins et le placebo. Can. Psychiat. Ass. J., 1975, **26**, 61-66

101. Greenblatt, M. Controls in clinical research. Clin. Pharmacol. Ther., 1964, 6 (2), 864-869

102. Huskisson, E.C. and Wojtulewski, J.A. Measurement of side effects of drugs. Br. Med. J., 1974, 2, 698-699

103. Ciccolunghi, S.N. and Chaudri, H.A. A methodological study of some factors influencing the reporting of symptoms. J. Clin. Pharmacol., 1975, July, 496-505

104. Lasagna, L. Bias in the elucidation of subjective side effects. Br. J. Clin. Pharmacol., 1981, 11, 111S-113S

105. New Zealand Hypertension Study Group. A multicentre open trial of labetalol in New Zealand. Br. J. Clin. Pharmacol., 1979, 179S-182S

106. Pessayre, D. and Benhamou, J.-P. 'Est-il possible et souhaitable de détecter l'hépatotoxicité d'un médicament avant sa commercialisation'. Gastroenterol. Clin. Biol., 1981, **5**, 560-563

107. Bulpitt, C.J. Quality of life in hypertensive patients. In Hypertensive Cardiovascular Disease: Pathophysiology and Treatment (ed. A. Amory), Martinus Nijhoff, The Hague, 1982

108. Jachuk, S.J., Brierley, H., Jachuk, S. and Willcox, P.M. The effect of hypotensive drugs on the quality of life. J. R. Coll. Gen. Pract., 1982, **32**, 103-105

109. Sengupta, R.P., Chin, J.S.P. and Brierley, H. Quality of survival following direct surgery for anterior communicating artery aneurysm. J. Neurosurg., 1975, **43**, 58-64

Chapter 3

110. Karch, F.E., Smith, C.L., Keizner, B., Mazzulo, J.M., Weintraub, M. and Lasagna, L. Adverse drug reactions - a

matter of opinion. Clin. Pharmacol. Ther., 1976, **19** (S, Pt 1), 489-492

111. Blanc, S., Leuenberger, P., Berger, J.-P., Brooks, E.M. and Schelling, J.-L. Judgment of trained observers on adverse drug reactions. Clin. Pharmacol. Ther., 1979, **25** (3), 493-498

112. Koch-Weser, J., Sellers, E.M. and Zacest, R. The ambiguity of adverse drug reactions. Eur. J. Clin. Pharmacol., 1977, **11**, 75-78

113. Berger, J.P., Haller, E., Blanc, S., Brooks, E.M. and Schelling, J.-L. Quelques facteurs intervenant dans les réactions adverses médicamenteuses. Schweiz. Med. Wochenschr. 1975, **105** (50), 1706-1708

114. Dangoumau, J., Begaud, B., Boisseau, A. and Albin, H. Les effets indésirables des médicaments. Diagnostics comparés de clinicians et pharmacoloques cliniciens. Nouv. Presse Med., 1980, 9 (23), 1607-1609

115. Kramer, M.S. Difficulties in assessing the adverse effects of drugs. Br. J. Clin. Pharmacol., 1981, **11**, 105S-110S

116. Dangoumau, J., Evreux, J.-C. and Jouglard, J. Méthode d'imputabilité des effets indésirables des médicaments. Thérapie, 1978, **33**, 373-381

117. Begaud, B., Boisseau, A., Albin, H. and Dangoumau, J. Imputabilité des effets indesirables des médicaments. Etude de 194 observations. Thérapie, 1978, **33**, 383-389

118. Karch, F.E. and Lasagna, L. Toward the operational identification of adverse drug reactions. Clin. Pharmacol. Ther., 1977, 21 (3), 247-253

119. Lapedes, D.N. (Ed.). Dictionary of Scientific and Technical Terms, McGraw-Hill, 1978

120. Irey, N.S. Tissue reactions to drugs. Am. J. Pathol., 1976, 82 (3), 617-647

121. Irey, N.S. Diagnostic problems in drug-induced diseases. In Drug-induced Diseases, Vol. 4 (ed. L. Meyler and H. Pek), Excerpta Medica, Amsterdam, 1972, pp.1-24

122. Farina, J.C., Krupp, P. and Tobler, H.J. Computer tools in spontaneous reporting of adverse drug reactions - A multinational approach. In Computer Aid to Drug Therapy and to Drug Monitoring (ed. Ducrot et al.), North-Holland, 1978, pp.117-123

123. Père, J.C., Begaud, B., Albin, H. and Dangoumau, J. Effets indésirables non-décrits de l'observation aux données de la litérature. Thérapie, 1981, **36**, 237-240

124. Weber, J.C.P. Storage and retrieval of data on adverse reactions to drugs. Interphex Symposium, Brighton, 10-13 June 1980

125. Jones, J.K. Revised causality algorithm, November 1980. Procedural Manual for handling drug experience reports, FDA

126. Hutchinson, T.A., Leventhal, J.M., Kramer, M.S., Karch, F.E., Lipman, A.G. and Feinstein, A.R. An algorithm for the operational assessment of adverse drug reactions, II:

Demonstration of reproducibility and validity. J.A.M.A., 1979, **242** (7), 633-638

127. Leventhal, J.M., Hutchinson, T.A., Kramer, M.S. and Feinstein, A.R. An algorithm for the operational assessment of adverse drug reactions, III: Results of tests among clinicians. J.A.M.A., 1979, **242** (18), 1991-1994

128. Venulet, J., Ciucci, A. and Berneker, G.C. Standardized assessment of drug-adverse reaction associations - rationale and experience. Int. J. Clin. Pharmacol. Ther. Toxicol., 1980, **18** (9), 381-388

129. Naranjo, C.A., Busto, U., Sellers, E.M. et al. A method for estimating the probability of adverse drug reactions. Clin. Pharmacol. Ther., 1981, **30**, 239-245

130. Busto, U., Naranjo, C.A. and Sellers, E.M. Comparison of two recently published algorithms for assessing the probability of adverse drug reactions. Br. J. Clin. Pharmacol., 1982, **13**, 112-117

131. Emanueli, A. and Sacchetti, G. An algorithm for the classification of untoward events in large scale clinical trials. In Agents and Actions, Vol. 7, Berkhäuser Verlag, Basle, 1980, pp.318-322

132. Report of Suspected Adverse Drug Reactions No. 4. Australian Government Publication Service, Canberra, 1978, p.v

133. Venning, G.R. Validity of anecdotal reports of suspected adverse drug reactions and the problems of false alarms. Br. Med. J., 1982, **284**, 249

134. Maistrello, I., Grassi, G., Bertolino, A., Valerio, P., Pistollato, G. and Soverini, S. Unwanted symptoms in depressed patients treated with viloxazine: an algorithm for identification of illness-related symptoms. Eur. J. Clin. Pharmacol., 1983, 24 Feb., 277-281

135. Dangoumau, J., Begaud, B., Boisseau, A. and Albin, H. Méthodes d'identification et d'imputabilité des effets indesirables des médicaments. Thérapie, 1980, **35**, 287-292

136. Leroy, O., Begaud, B., Dangoumau, J., Peytour, P. and Salamon, R. Etude comparative de quatre méthodes d'imputabilité. Thérapie, 1981, **36**, 223-227

137. Begaud, B., Boisseau, A., Albin, H. and Dangoumau, J. Comparaison de quatre méthodes d'imputabilité des effets indesirables des médicaments. Thérapie, 1981, **31** (1), 65-70

138. Begaud, B., Haramburu, F., Père, J.C. and Dangoumau, J. Les critères d'imputabilité confrontés à la pratique à propos de 1000 observations. Thérapie, 1982, **37**, 415-420

139. Salamon, R. and Peytour, P. Recherche du poids des critères dans un algorithme d'imputabilité. Thérapie, 1981, **36**, 229-231

140. Dangoumau, J., Begaud, B., Père, J.C. and Albin, H. De l'imputabilité originelle à l'imputabilité terminal. Thérapie, 1981, **361**, 219-227

141. Boisseau, A., Begaud, B., Albin, H. and Dangoumau, J. Réevaluation du diagnostic d'effets indésirables des

médicaments avec un recul de six mois. Thérapie, 1980, **35**, 577-580

142. Dangoumau, J., Begaud, B., Boisseau, A. and Albin, H. Méthodes d'identification de l'imputabilité des effets indesirables des médicaments. L'effect indesirable, une realité fuyante? Thérapie, 1980, **35**, 287-292

143. Prichard, B.N.C. Hypotensive action of Pronethalol. Br. Med. J., 1964, **1**, 1227-1228

144. Baumelou, A. and Legrain, M. Medical nephrectomy with anti-inflammatory non-steroidal drugs. Br. Med. J., 1982, **284**, 234

145. Gagnon, M.-A. Subjective phenomena in drug trials. Int. J. Clin. Pharmacol., 1977, **15** (4), 155-160

146. McPherson, K., Healey, M.J.R., Flynn, F.V. and Piper, K.A.J. The effect of age, sex and other factors on blood chemistry in health. Clin. Chim. Acta, 1978, **84**, 373-397

147. Presentation of Observed Values. Part 6: The Theory of Reference Values, I.F.C.C. Document 1982 (Stages 1 and 2), 1982, **7**, 27

148. Ciccolunghi, S.M., Fowler, P.D. and Chaudri, M.J. Interpretation of haematological and biochemical laboratory data in large-scale multicentre clinical trials. J. Clin. Pharmacol., 1979, **19**, 302-312

149. Pitts, N.E. Prazosin -- Evaluation of a New Hypertensive Agent, International Congress Series No. 331, Excerpta Medica, Amsterdam, 1974, p.159

Chapter 4

150. Cardon, P.V., Dommel, F.W. and Trumble, R.R. Injuries to research subjects - a survey of investigators. New Engl. J. Med., 1976, **295**, 650-654

151. Zarafonetes, C.J.D. et al. Clinically significant adverse events in a Phase 1 testing program. Clin. Pharmacol. Ther., 1978, **24** (2), 127-132

152. Kinney, E.L., Trautman, J., Gold, J.A., Vesell, E.S. and Zelis, R. Underrepresentation of women in new drug trials: ramification and remedies. Ann. Intern. Med., 1981, **915** (5), 560-563

153. General Considerations for the Clinical Evaluation of Drugs. Health, Education and Welfare (F.D.A), 77-3040, Sept. 1977, p.10

154. Hollister, L.E. Prediction of therapeutic uses of psycho-therapeutic drugs from experience with normal volunteers. Clin. Pharmacol. Ther., 1972, **13** (2), 803-808

155. Azarnoff, D.L. Physiologic factors in selecting human volunteers for drug studies. Clin. Pharmacol. Ther., 1972, **13** (3), Pt 2, 796-802

156. Lasagna, L. and Von Felsinger, J.M. The volunteer subject. Res. Sci., 1954, **126**, 359-361

157. Oater, J.A. A scientific rationale for choosing patients rather than normal subjects for Phase 1 studies. Clin. Pharmacol. Ther., 1972, **13** (5), Pt 2, 809-811

158. Weissman, L. Multiple dose Phase 1 trials. Normal volunteers or patients: one viewpoint. J. Clin. Pharmacol., 1981, 21, 385-387

159. Clinical Trials Unit, Department of Pharmacology and Therapeutics, London Hospital Medical College. Aide-memoire for preparing clinical trial protocols. Br. Med. J., 1977, 21 May, 1323-1324

160. Spriet, A. and Simon, P. Questions à se poser pour vérifier un protocole d'essai thérapeutique avant d'entreprendre l'éxécution. Thérapie, 1977, 32, 633-642

161. Offerhaus, L. Guidelines for evaluation of antihypertensive drugs in man. Eur. J. Clin. Pharmacol., 1979, 16, 427-430

162. Guidelines for Preclinical and Clinical Testing of New Medicinal Products, Part 2 - Investigations in Man. Ass. Br. Pharm. Ind., 1977, p.13

163. Sackett, D.L. and Gent. M. Controversy in counting and attributing events in clinical trials. New Engl. J. Med., 1979, 301 (26), 1410-1412

164. De Metz, D., Friedman, L. and Furberg, C. Counting events in clinical trials. New Engl. J. Med., 1980, 302 (16), 924-925

165. May, G.S., De Metz, D.L., Friedman, L.M., Furberg, C. and Passamani, E. The randomised clinical trial: bias in analysis. Circulation, 1981, 64 (4), 669-673

166. Cancer Research Campaign Working Party. Trials and tribulations: thoughts on the organisation of multicentre clinical studies. Br. Med. J., 1980, 281, 918-920

167. Leganière, S. and Brion, P. Clinical trials: incomplete reporting of side effects. Curr. Ther. Res., 1979, 25 (6), 743-746

168. Halsey, J.P. and Cardoe, N. Benoxaprofen side effects profile in 300 patients. Br. Med. J., 1982, 284, 1365-1368

169. Idänpään-Meikkilä, J. A review of Safety Information Obtained from Phase I, II and III Clinical Investigation of Sixteen Selected Drugs. US Dept of Health and Human Services, June 1983

170. Hemminki, E. Study of information submitted by drug companies to licensing authorities. Br. Med. J., 1980, 22 March, 833-836

171. Azarnoff, D.L., Abrams, W.B., Cuttner, J., Hewitt, W.L. and Hartman, M. Phase III investigations. Clin. Pharmacol. Ther., 1975, 18 (5) Pt 2, 650-652

172. Laganière, S. and Brion, P. Clinical trials: incomplete reporting of side effects. Curr. Ther. Res., 1979, 25 (6), 743-746

173. Hibberd, P.L. and Meadows, A.J. Information contained in clinical trial reports. J. Inform. Sci., 1980, 2, 169-172

174. Huskisson, E.C. Good and bad clinical trials: a checklist. J. Hosp. Pharm., 1973, June, July, Aug

175. Herxheimer, A. and Lionel, N.D.W. Assessing reports of therapeutic trials. Proc. Br. Pharm. Soc., 1970, April, 204P-205P

176. Burley, D.M. and Binns, T.B. Erroneous adverse reaction reports. Lancet, 1976, 29 May, 1193

177. Venulet, J., Blattner, R., Von Bülow, J. and Berneker, G.C. How good are articles on adverse drug reactions? Br. Med. J., 1982, **284**, 252-254

178. Venning, G.R. Validity of anecdotal reports of suspected adverse reactions: the problem of false alarms. Br. Med. J., 1982, **284**, 249-252

179. Albin, H., Begaud, B., Boisseau, A. and Dangoumau, J. Validation des publications d'effets indésirables par une méthode d'imputabilité. Thérapie, 1980, **33**, 511-536

180. Herxheimer, A. and Lionel, N.D.W. Minimum information needed by prescriber, Br. Med. J., 1978, **2**, 1129-1132

Chapter 5

181. Deitch, R. Adverse reactions to drugs. Lancet, 1980, 17 May, 1095

182. Harrow, D.W.G., Griffiths, K. and Shanks, R.G. Debendox and congenital malformations in Northern Ireland. Br. Med. J., 1980, **281**, 1274-1381

183. Anon. Pertussis vaccine. Br. Med. J., 1981, **22** (6276), 1563

184. Anon. Crying wolf on drug safety. Br. Med. J., 1982, **284** (6311), 219

185. Anon. Hunting rare adverse drug reactions. Br. Med. J., 1981, **282**, 342-343

186. Martys, C.R. Adverse reactions to drugs in general practice. Br. Med. J., 1979, **2**, 1194-1197

187. Gifford, L.M., Aeugle, M.E., Myerson, R.N. and Tannenbaum, P.J. Cimetidine postmarket surveillance program. J.A.M.A., 1980, **243** (15), 1532

188. Rawlins, M.D. and Dollery, C.T. Postmarketing surveillance of adverse reactions to new medicines. Medico-pharmaceutical Forum Publication No. 7, 1977

189. O'Neill, R. Appendix 1 of Reference 169

190. Boman, G. The nordic countries. In Monitoring for Drug Safety (ed. W.H.W. Inman), M.T.P., 1980

191. Liljestrand. In Drug Induced Sufferings: Medical, Pharmaceutical and Legal Aspects (ed. T. Soda), Excerpta Medica, Amsterdam, 1980, p.234

192. Inman, W.H.W. and Mustrin, W.W. Jaundice after repeated exposure to halothane: an analysis of reports to the Committee on Safety of Medicines. Br. Med. J., 1974, **1**, 5

193. Inman, W.H.W. and Vessey, M.P. Investigation of deaths from pulmonary coronary and cerebral thrombosis and embolism in women of childbearing age. Br. Med. J., 1968, **2**, 193-199

194. Inman, W.H.W., Vessey, M.P., Westerholm, B. and Engelind, A. Thromboembolic disease and the steroidal content of oral contraceptives. Br. Med. J., 1970, **2**, 203

195. Cahal, D.A. Adverse reactions to nalidixic acid. Lancet, 1965 **ii**, 441

196. Wade, G.L. In Adverse Drug Reactions (ed. D.J. Richards and R.K. Rondel), Churchill Livingstone, 1972, p.52

197. Anon. How the yellow card system might be improved. Pharm. J., 1983, 6 Aug., 160

198. Griffin, J.P. Postmarketing surveillance of licensed medicinal and other products. Health Trends, 1981, 13, 87

199. Inman, W.H.W. and Rawson, N.S.B. Erythromycin estolate and jaundice. Br. Med. J., 1983, 286, 1954-1955

200. Wiholm, B.E., Agenäs, I. and Boethius, G. Improving the evaluation of adverse drug reactions by use of drug utilisation and morbidity data. Proc. S.P.S., B.P.S., 5-6 July 1982, 596

201. Scrip, 1981, No.639, November, 1

202. Follath, F., Burkart, F. and Schweizer, W. Drug-induced pulmonary hypertension. Br. Med. J., 1971, 1, 265

203. Fraumeni, J.F. Bone marrow depression induced by chloramphenicol and phenylbutazone. J.A.M.A., 1967, 20 (1), 828

204. Constant, K.W., Worlledge, S., Dollery, C.T. and Breckenridge, A. Methyl Dopa and haemolytic anaemia. Lancet, 1966, 22 January, 201

205. Rich, M.L., Rittehof, R.J. and Hoffmann, R.J. A fatal case of aplastic anaemia following chloramphenicol (chloromycetin) therapy. Ann. Intern. Med., 1950, 33, 1459-1467

206. Wright, P.E. Skin reaction to practolol. Br. Med. J., 1974, 2, 560

207. Dollery, C.T. and Rawlins, M.D. Monitoring adverse reactions to drugs. Br. Med. J., 1977, 1, 96-97

208. Lawson, D.H. and Henry, D.A. Monitoring adverse reactions to new drugs: restricted release or monitored release. Br. Med. J., 1977, 1, 691-692

209. Inman, W.H.W. Recorded release: a proposal for postmarketing surveillance of new drugs. Paper read at Symposium on Drug Control in General Practice, June 1977

210. Wilson, A.B. Postmarketing surveillance of adverse reactions to new medicines. Br. Med. J., 1977, 2, 1001-1003

211. Walden, R.J. and Prichard, B.N.C. Postmarketing drug surveillance. Br. J. Clin. Pharmacol., 1978, 6, 191-192

212. C.S.M. Suggestions for monitoring adverse drug reactions. Pharm. J., 1977, 9 July, 30-31

213. Anon. New strategies for drug monitoring. Br. Med. J., 1977, 1, 861

214. Moir, D.C. Drug monitoring. Br. Med. J., 1981, 282, 632

215. Skegg, D.C.G. Adverse reaction monitoring in the future. In Pharmaceutical Medicine (ed. N. McLeod), Churchill Livingstone

216. Lawson, D.H. Detection of drug-induced disease. Br. J. Clin. Pharmacol., 1979, 7, 13-18

217. Spriet-Pourra, C. Different approaches of postmarketing surveillance: their realism and interest. Curr. Ther. Res., 1979, 25 (2)

218. Inman, W.H.W. Recorded release. In Drug Monitoring (ed. F.H. Gross and W.H.W. Inman), Academic Press, 1977

219. Heaseman, M.A. and Lipworth, L. Accuracy of Certification of Cause of Death. Studies on Medical and Population Subjects, 1966, No. 20, H.M.S.O.

220. Rose, G. Bias. Br. J. Clin. Pharmacol., 1982, 13, 157-162

221. Finney, D.J. The design and logic of a monitor of drug use. J. Chron. Dis., 1965, 18, 77-98

222. Skegg, D.C.G. Medical Record Linkage. In Monitoring for Drug Safety (ed. W.H.W. Inman), M.T.P.

223. Ichänpään-Heikkila, J. Population monitoring: medical linkage for drug safety surveillance. In Drug Monitoring (ed. F.H. Gross and W.H.W. Inman), Academic Press, 1977

224. Miller, R.R. Comprehensive prospective drug surveillance - A report from the Boston Collaborative Drug Surveillance Program. Pharm. Weekbl., 1974, 109, 461-481

225. Moir, D.C. Intensive monitoring in hospital, II: The Aberdeen-Dundee System. In Monitoring for Drug Safety (ed. W.H.W. Inman), M.T.P.

226. Friedman, G.O., Collen, M.F., Harris, L.E., Van Brunt, E.E. and Davis, L.S. Experience in monitoring drug reactions in outpatients - The Kaiser-Permanente Drug Monitoring System. J.A.M.A., 1971, 217 (5), 567-572

227. Crombie, I.K. Dundee Record Linkage Study. In Monitoring for Adverse Drug Reactions (ed. S. Walker and A. Goldberg), M.T.P., 1984

228. Jones, J.K. Postmarketing surveillance. An FDA perspective presented at the annual Society for Clinical Pharmacology and Therapeutic Postgraduate Course, New Orleans, 1981

229. Title XIX's Medicaid Management Information System as a Data Resource for Conducting Postmarketing Surveillance Studies and Evaluation of this Data Base for Drug Utilization Studies. Principal Investigators, L. Moise and A. Leroy. Health Information Design Inc. Contract Nos. 223-80-3026, 223-78-3018

230. Scrip. 1982, 24 February, 670

231. Tukey, J.W. Some thoughts on clinical trials, especially problems of multiplicity. Science, 1977, 198, 679-684

232. Anon. Benoxaprofen photosensitivity - a test for prescription monitoring. Lancet, 1982, 3 April, 811

233. Lawson, D.H. Postmarketing surveillance in U.K.: a study of cimetidine recipients. In Drug Safety and Controversies (ed. M. Auriche, J. Burk and J. Duchier, Pergamon Press, 1981

234. Colin-Jones, D.G., Langman, M.J.S., Lawson, D.H. and Vessey, M.P. Postmarketing surveillance. In Cimetidine in the 80s (ed. J.H. Baron), Churchill Livingstone, 1981

235. Colin-Jones, D.G., Langman, M.J.S., Lawson, D.H. and Vessey, M.P. Postmarketing surveillance of the safety of cimetidine. 12 monthly mortality report. Br. Med. J., 1983, 286, 1713-1716

236. Drury, M. and Hull, F.M. Prospective monitoring for adverse reactions to drugs in general practice. Br. Med. J., 1981, 283, 1305

237. Horowitz, R. and Feinstein, A.R. The application of therapeutic trial principles to improve the design of epidemiological

research – a case control study suggesting that anticoagulants reduce mortality in patients with myocardial infarction. J. Chron. Dis., 1981, **34**, 575-581

238.   Mantel, N. and Haenzell, W. Statistical aspects of the analysis of data from retrospective studies of disease. J. Natl Cancer Inst., 1959, **22** (4), 719-748

239.   Sackett, D.L. Bias in analytical research. J. Chron. Dis., 1979, **32**, 51-63

240.   Smith, M.W. The case control or retrospective study: in retrospect. J. Clin. Pharmacol., 1981, **21**, 269-274

241.   Horowitz, R.I. and Feinstein, A.R. The problem of proto-pathic bias in case control studies. Am. J. Med., 1980, **68**, 255-258

242.   Spriet-Pourra, C. Postmarketing surveillance by the drug industry. Discussion on postmarketing surveillance of drug effects organised by the Drug Surveillance Research Unit on behalf of the European Community, Southampton, 8-10 April, 1981

243.   Pryor, J.P. and Castle, W.M. Peyronie's disease associated with chronic degenerative arterial disease and not with beta-adrenoceptor blocking agents. Lancet, 1982, 17 April, 917

244.   Jick, H. Cohorts from data banks. In Drug Safety and Controversies (ed. M. Auriche, J. Burk and J. Duchier), Pergamon Press, 1981

245.   Westlin, W.E., Cuddihy, R.V., Bursik, R.J., Seifert, B.G. and Koelle, J.G. One method for the systematic evaluation of adverse drug experience data within a pharmaceutical firm. Methods Inf. Med., 1977, **16** (4), 240-241

246.   Castle, W.M. Placing adverse reaction reports in perspective. In Proceedings 7th Annual Conference of A.I.O.P.I., 1980, pp.48-50

247.   Begaud, B., Pére, J.-C. and Dangoumau, J. Mise en oeuvre d'une critére. La bibliographie. Thérapie, 1981, **36**, 233-236

248.   Sullman, S.F. A resumé of the pharmaceutical industry's experience with monitored release. In Post-marketing Surveil-lance of Adverse Reactions to New Medicines. Medico-Pharma-ceutical Forum, Publication No. 7, 1977

249.   A.B.P.I. (Personal communication)

250.   Rossi, A.C., Knapp, D.E., Anello, C., O'Neill, R.T., Grahan, C.F., Mendelis, P.S. and Stomley, G.R. Discovery of adverse reactions. A comparison of selected Phase IV studies, with spontaneous reporting methods. J.A.M.A., 1983, **249**, 2226-2228

251.   Anello, C. The use, design and limitations of selected Phase IV studies in the USA. Droit et Pharmacie Essais Clinique Post Marketing, 1983, Vol. III

252.   Perry-Evans, D. Monitoring adverse reactions to drugs. M.D. Thesis, University of London, 1976

253.   Stephens, M.D.B. Monitoring for Adverse Drug Reactions. A Workshop under the Auspices of the UK Centre for Medicines Research, M.T.P., 1984

254. Code of practice for the clinical assessment of licensed medicinal products in general practice. Br. Med. J., 1983, **286**, 1295-1297

255. Bruppacher, R. Dual purpose of inpatient drug monitoring by physicians in two teaching hospitals in Berne. In Computer Aid to Drug Therapy and Drug Monitoring, Chapter 6 (ed. Ducrot et al.), North-Holland, 1978

256. Venulet, J., Berneker, G.C. and Ciucci, A. (Eds). Assessing Causes of Adverse Drug Reaction, Academic Press, 1982

257. Loupi, E., Ponchon, A., Ventre, J.J., Descotes, S.J. and Evreux, J.-Cl. La réadministration (rechallenge) est-elle necessaire a une imputabilité maximale? (Valeur comparée dans sept méthodes d'imputabilité) Cinquieme Journée Françaises de Pharmacovigilance, 1983

258. Hammond, K.R. and Joyce, C.R.B. Psychological influences on human judgement, especially of adverse reactions. In Drug Monitoring (ed. F.M. Gross and W.H.W. Inman), Academic Press, 1977, p.272

259. Stephens, M.D.B. Deliberate drug rechallenge. Hum. Toxicol., 1983, 2, 573-577

260. Klatskin, G. and Kimberg, D.V. Recurrent hepatitis attributable to halothane sensitization in an anaesthetist. New Engl. J. Med., 1969, **280** (10), 515-522

261. Douglas, J.G., Munro, J.F., Kitchin, A.H., Muir, A.L. and Proudfoot, A.T. Pulmonary hypertension and fenfluramine. Br. Med. J., 1981, **283**, 881-883

262. Mathison, D.A. and Stevenson, D.D. Hypersensitivity to non-steroidal anti-inflammatory drugs. Indications and methods for oral rechallenges. J. Allergy Clin. Immunol., 1979, **64** (6), 669-674

263. Baumelou, A. Les etudes de Phase IV en France: Analyse des differentes commissions de la direction de la pharmacie et du medicament. Essais Clinique Post-marketing Vol. III, Chapter 8, Droit et Pharmacie, Paris, Sept., 1983

264. Jones, J.K. Criteria for journal reports of suspected adverse drug reactions. Clin. Pharm., 1982, 1, 554-555

265. Rogers, M.L. National abstracts: U.K. hospital pharmacists collaborative computerised database. In The Impact of Computer Technology on Drug Information (ed. P. Morrell and S.G. Johansson), North-Holland, 1982, pp.187-188

266. Simkins, M.A. A comparison of databases for retrieving references to the literature on drugs. Information Processing and Management, 1977, 13, 141-153

267. Anon. Adverse Drug Reactions Advisory Committee Report for 1978. Med. J. Aust., 1980, 1, 207-208

268. Morley, D. CAIRS. In Minis, Micros and Terminals for Libraries and Information Services (ed. Gilchrist), Haydon, 1981, pp.78-89

269. Helling, M. Use of computers in drug monitoring. In Monitoring for Drug Safety (ed. W.H.W. Inman), 1980, M.T.P.. pp/141-164

270. Wright, P. and Haybittle, J. Design of forms for clinical trials (1). Br. Med. J., 1979, 2, 529-530
271. Idem, 1979, 2, 590-592
272. Idem, 1979, 2, 650-651
273. Rycroft, D. and Smith, D.E. Provision of poisons and safety data. Aslib Proc., 1980, 32 (5), 235-240
274. Ravenscroft, T. and Smith, D.E. The development of Clindata. A clinical trial data management system. J. Inf. Sci., 1981, 3, 129-136
275. National Adverse Drug Reaction Directory COSTART (Coding Symbols for Thesaurus of Adverse Reaction Terms), US Dept of Health, Education and Welfare, F.D.A.
276. W.H.O. International Classification of Diseases. Manual of the International Statistics Classification of Diseases, Injuries and Causes of Death. Vol. 1 and Vol. 2, Alphabetical index, 9th revision (1975), HMSO, 1977
277. National Library of Medicine, Medical Subject Headings (MeSH). Annotated alphabetical list, 1984
278. Oxmis Problem Codes (ed. J. Perry), Oxmis Publications, Oxford, 1978
279. Perry, J. A primary care morbidity code based on the international classification of diseases. In Medical Data Processing (ed. M. Laudet, J. Anderson and F. Bregon), Taylor and Francis, 1976, pp.719-725
280. Cote, R.A. (ed.). Systematised Nomenclature of Medicine (SNOMED). Vol. I, 2nd edn, College of American Pathologists, 1979 (Numeric index)
281. Idem. Vol. II, 2nd edn, College of American Pathologists, 1979 (Alphabetic index)
282. Cote, R.A. and Robboy, S. Progress in medical information management. Systematised Nomenclature of Medicine (SNOMED). J.A.M.A., 1980, 243, 756-762
283. Anon. International monitoring of adverse reactions to drugs. Adverse reaction terminology 1980. Collaborating Centre for International Drug Monitoring, Uppsala, Sweden
284. Monthly Index of Medical Specialties (MIMS). Haymarket Publishing, London (published monthly)
285. British National Formulary, Number 6, 1983. Pharmaceutical Press, London (updated 6-monthly)
286. Dendy, P.R. Indexing Medicines for Monitoring Adverse Reactions. Oxford Drug Monitoring Conference - Workshop on Drug Information System, 1977. Oxford Community Health Project, A1-A4
287. Dunleavy, J. and Perry, J. Appendix B. Oxmis problem codes and drug codes. Idem, B24-B25 .

Chapter 9

288. Hansson, O. The voice of the consumer. In Drug Induced Sufferings. Medical, Pharmaceutical and Legal Aspects (ed. T. Soda), Excerpta Medica, Amsterdam, 1980, p.20

289. Nagarro, K., Onishi, Y. and Ozaki, J. Comparison of the drug affairs acts of different countries and problems of the amendment of the Japanese Drug Affairs Act in session. In Drug Induced Sufferings: Medical, Pharmaceutical and Legal Aspects (ed. T. Soda), Excerpta Medica, Amsterdam, 1980, p.281

290. Silverman, M. and Lydecker, M. Disclosures of hazards in international drug promotion. In Drug Induced Sufferings: Medical, Pharmaceutical and Legal Aspects (ed. T. Soda), Excerpta Medica, Amsterdam, 1980, pp.359-364

291. Shapiro, S. General discussion. In Drug Monitoring (ed. F.H. Gross and W.H.W. Inman), Academic Press, 1977, p.153

292. Temple, R. General discussion. In Drug Monitoring (ed. F.H. Gross and W.H.W. Inman), Academic Press, 1977, p.156

293. Fülgraff, G. General discussion. In Drug Monitoring (ed. F.H. Gross and W.H.W. Inman), Academic Press, 1977, p.156

294. Scrip, No 831, Sept. 21 1983, 12; No 854, Dec. 12, 1983, 5

295. Turner, P. Future trends in pharmaceutical medicine. In Pharmaceutical Medicine (ed. N. Macleod), Churchill Livingstone, 1978, p.156

Index*

*The terms 'ADR' and 'adverse event' have been used in their
true sense in this index, as throughout the text. The reader
who is unfamiliar with the subject is advised to look under
both headings when consulting the index.